THE YEAR OF THE ZEBRA

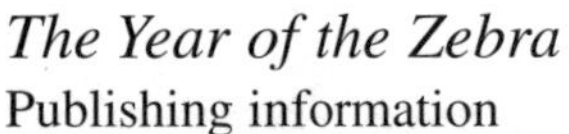

The Year of the Zebra
Publishing information

Photographs provided by Scott Mitchell and John Thomas Photography Rock Island, Illinois. Composite family picture created by Nicholsons' Racine, Wisconsin.

Cover design and book layout by Greg Blair of Silverline Design Studios, Milwaukee, Wisconsin.

*The entire purchase price of this book will be donated
to scholarships in Keith's memory.*

ISBN 0-966-15090-2

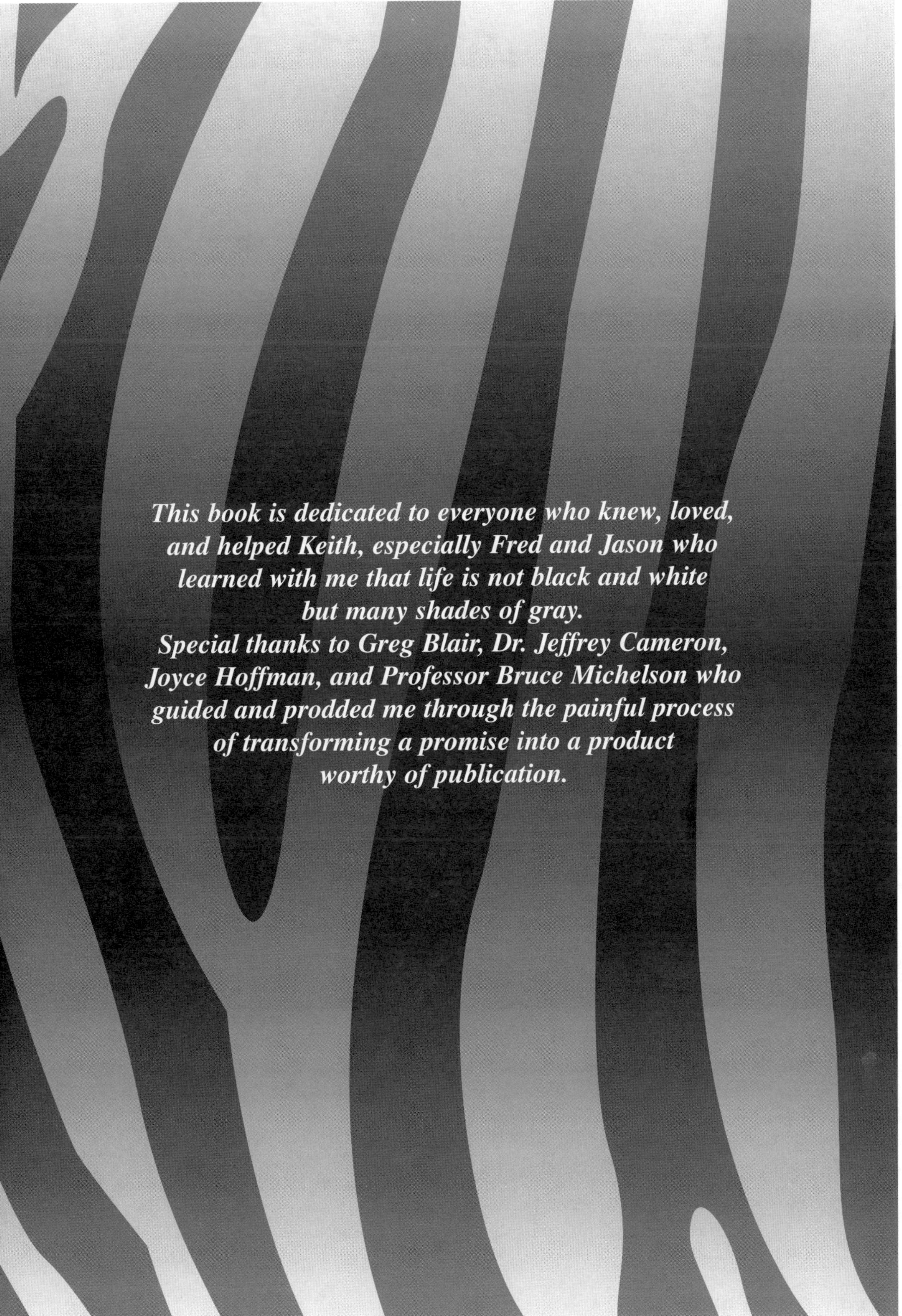

This book is dedicated to everyone who knew, loved,
and helped Keith, especially Fred and Jason who
learned with me that life is not black and white
but many shades of gray.
Special thanks to Greg Blair, Dr. Jeffrey Cameron,
Joyce Hoffman, and Professor Bruce Michelson who
guided and prodded me through the painful process
of transforming a promise into a product
worthy of publication.

by Jeffrey S. Cameron, MD

I first met Keith Kelroy when he came to Sacred Heart Rehabilitation Institute in Milwaukee for outpatient therapy in late October of 1995. He was referred to me to supervise his progress in therapy. Keith was a handsome, physically fit, All-American looking young man, with a good sense of humor, a strong enthusiasm for therapy, and an intelligence that was obvious in spite of his mild word-finding difficulty. He had a right-sided weakness that had occurred during a brain biopsy that had been done to determine the cause of two large cystic masses that had been found in his brain on an MRI scan. Based on the appearance of his MRI, his doctors had strongly suspected either cancer or an infection, and needed to perform the biopsy to obtain a diagnosis; the finding of only demyelination was a surprise.

Demyelination refers to a disruption of the myelin sheath that surrounds the axons (the long thin extensions that connect to other cells) of nerve cells and allows for the rapid transmission of an electric signal. Disruption of the myelin sheath interferes with nerve cell communication. Demyelination is a hallmark of Multiple Sclerosis, but it can also be seen in many other conditions. This was such an unusual initial presentation for Multiple Sclerosis, that in spite of the finding of demyelination, I questioned the diagnosis. I was very excited when one of the therapists working with Keith found an article describing 31 cases of large, tumor-like demyelinating lesions. This article stated that 90% of these patients never developed any additional lesions, and it proposed that these cases represented an intermediate entity between Multiple Sclerosis and another condition. This article gave us all hope that if Keith could only recover from this episode of demyelination, maybe his ordeal would be over.

Keith was initially placed on high dose steroids in an attempt to halt the demyelinating process, but by the time he saw me he had started on a tapering schedule. At our first meeting Keith indicated that his right sided weakness had seemed a little worse over the last few days, so his doctors in Madison had just increased his oral steroid dose back to his previous level. Over the next few days he continued to lose strength to the point where he could barely walk, and, after conferring with his neurologist in Madison, I ended up having to admit Keith to the hospital again for intravenous steroids. This decline in function turned out to be the first of what would prove to be many relapses for Keith. As he would continually improve only to worsen again, I developed a special relationship with Keith and his family. Although primary treatment of Keith's condition was outside my realm of practice as a rehabilitation physician, I helped Keith and his family obtain additional medical opinions and tried to help them process the advice they were getting. Despite the many setbacks he encountered in his last year of life, Keith never lost his hopefulness about the future, his drive and determination to get better, his competitiveness, his sense of humor, his faith, or his generosity of spirit.

About a month before he died, Keith became comatose with a high blood ammonia level, and I visited him and his mom in the hospital. When Karen told me the doctors were thinking that a rare metabolic abnormality might be the cause of the high ammonia in response to one of his medications, I remarked to her that, if true, it would mean Keith had two "zebra" diagnoses, and then explained to her what I meant by a "zebra." In an attempt to counteract the tendency of medical students to diagnose rare and exotic illnesses they are taught that common things happen commonly, using the following illustration: suppose you hear hoofbeats on the street outside your window - while it is possible they will belong to a zebra, it is far more likely they belong to a horse. Accordingly, when medical students or physicians encounter highly unusual cases, they sometimes refer to these cases as "zebras." This concept of Keith's case being a "zebra" resonated with Karen, and she incorporated it into the title of this book.

Keith's journal entries by themselves would be an engrossing and moving account of the last year of his life. However, the addition of Karen's entries, giving us the family's perspective adds tremendously to the emotional power and drama of this book.

<u>The Year of the Zebra</u> is a compelling true story of a remarkable young man's battle against a rare incurable illness. It will leave the reader inspired by the love, faith, and courage of the entire Kelroy family. You will read the four promises Karen made to Keith before he died. With the writing of this book, Karen has fulfilled her promises to her son.

The week before my 24 year old son died I made him four promises. I promised Keith not to become bitter, to keep the faith, find happiness in life, and write this book. The painful fact Keith died makes this book significantly different from other motivational or inspirational books. Ours is a story of unanswered prayers for physical healing, of disappointment, and disillusionment, as well as a confirmation there is a personal God who offers hope during despair, gives an assurance Easter follows the Good Fridays of life, and provides for a happy ending.

You will meet Keith through his tapes, what others have written about him, and my biased perspective. He recorded much of his last several months of life on tapes labeled "Hell" with the intention of publishing his own journal, but with his death on August 12, 1996, that responsibility fell on me. You will also get to know Fred, Keith's dad, who is my best friend and husband of 27 years. In addition you will be introduced to Keith's best friend, his brother Jason, who made the year bearable for all of us. The setting will change often as Keith was in 10 hospitals in 11 months, each relocation based on physicians' decisions as a form of crisis intervention.

Hearing about answered prayer during our many crises was not always comforting. For while God was healing others so they could swim in water, if not walk on it, I often felt like I was drowning in a pool of sadness created by my own tears. For if I allowed myself to believe God loved those people so much that He healed them, the converse came naturally, He didn't really care about what was happening to our family. Initially sayings like "miracles happen to those who believe" were disconcerting because we never experienced any miraculous consistent physical healing and we are believers. However, while our hearts were set on the miracle of physical healing we were touched by God, and in the end experienced a miracle that was larger than life. A miracle that Keith and I would like to share with you. The easiest way for us to do that is to write in double entry journal form. Keith's entries come primarily from his recordings, while mine are from memories and feelings carved deep into a mother's heart. Before I begin the story, I would like to introduce you to Keith and our family by sharing a few of the hundreds of messages we received following his death.

"He was an extraordinary young man, and his loss diminishes us all."
Professor Bruce Michelson - University of Illinois at Urbana - Champaign

"Keith touched all who knew him with his sense of optimism and kindness."
Dr. Brian Weinshenker - Mayo Clinic - Rochester, Minnesota

"Keith showed a promising career with Quantum Chemical."
Ronald H. Yocum Chairman - President and Chief Executive Officer
Quantum Chemical Corporation

"Keith had an open, cheerful, and grateful approach to life's opportunities. What is more, his attitude was contagious...I could not help thinking then as I do now, of how proud you deserve to be for having raised such a thoughtful, warm, open, decent, fun-loving, and thoroughly admirable young man."
Dr. Richard W. Burkhardt - Director Campus Honors Program
University of Illinois

"Keith's family meant everything to him."
Susan Ganster - Marketing Manager, Injection Molding for Quantum

"I cannot imagine I will ever see more love, compassion, and caring between one family. You have taught me that there is truly nothing more important than family and showing your love to those most important to you."
Mike Buckholdt - Physical Therapist- Froedtert Hospital

It was three weeks after Keith's death when I put his first tape into my car tape deck and once again heard his voice which was the beginning of writing this book. As thoughts started to crystallize in my mind I realized he really began telling the story at the age of 17 when he wrote about how much our family meant to him. This is what Keith wrote in an application essay for his selection as a Chancellor Scholar at the University of Illinois which was an honor bestowed on 100 of the incoming class of 10,000 freshmen.

I am seventeen years old and only half a year away from leaving home. My childhood has ended and I will be setting off to make it on my own at the big university. Yet I know I always have something to fall back on. I will never really be all alone. My family has and will continue to always be there for me. I feel there is nothing more important than a good family. Without a doubt I have been blessed with one.

My parents have always stressed the importance of a closely knit family and I have accepted my family as an especially important part of my life also. Through family I have established my set of morals and values. It is from my parents that these have been created, and for them I am very thankful. My brother and I could have no better role models than in our parents. They have constantly, without fault, demonstrated and lived by values which any man would be proud to call his own. My parents live by the rules of loving, sharing, caring, and forgiving. These are only a few of the characteristics that lead me to believe I am blessed with a family second to none.

My parents have taught me to strive for the best and settle for nothing less. Whatever my best is it is good enough for them. Usually not for me, but always is good enough for them. When I succeed they are there to congratulate me. When I fall they are there to pick me up. My family has instilled in me the desire to succeed but to never walk over others in the process. They have taught me to be modest in winning and to hold my head high when losing. They are the people who have taught me to deal with success and live with failure.

I tend to believe I have turned out to be a pretty good person. I give the credit to my parents and my brother, for I am not always an easy person to raise or to live with. It is my family that has constantly straightened out my path through life. They give until they can give no more, and they never stop caring. I owe who I am to my family and for that I can never repay them. It is my family that is especially important to me. My family has always been there for me and they always will be. I can ask for no more. There is nothing more to ask for.

Those closing sentences took on greater meaning than I believe Keith ever intended. Keith brought more meaning and joy into our lives than I could ever describe. Forever would not have been long enough to spend with him nor a moment too brief for to be touched by Keith's love was to be changed forever, and indeed a priceless gift to all of us.

CHAPTER ONE

Trinity Hospital - Cudahy, Wisconsin

From the very beginning, Keith was on an accelerated course through life. His arrival June 14, 1972, was two weeks early and quick. He only gave us 90 minutes warning which was barely enough time to get to Trinity Hospital as it took us first time parents a little while to figure out I was actually in labor. His alertness in the hospital nursery was so unusual the nurses sent us on our way with the parting words "good luck," and that is exactly what we had for 23 years.

Keith was raised at 7527 Sylvan Drive, Caledonia, Wisconsin, the address of our first house. Religious reasons had brought us to the western shores of Lake Michigan. Fred was born and raised Catholic on a dairy farm seventy miles north of Milwaukee. St. John's Catholic Church is next to the farm. Ever since I was old enough to attend Sunday School I went to Trinity Lutheran Church in Madison which is seventy miles west of Milwaukee. It was there I made lifelong friends such as Kay and Penny. Kay was my college roommate at the University of Wisconsin-Oshkosh where I met Fred, and she pointed out there would be religious conflicts if I married him when she tacked "Luther Forever" to our door. Fred and I both had a solid faith foundation when we met, and enjoyed growing in our faith and love through the many campus Christian activities held at the Newman Center. We believed in the importance of being part of an active faith community, and we wanted our future children raised with a common faith. The problem was we couldn't agree on the common faith. In the end, with the help of my father, I decided I could worship within the Catholic setting as long as Fred agreed our children would be raised with an ecumenical spirit, exposed to both our spiritual backgrounds, and be allowed to determine their own house of worship free of the pressures we were facing. We had decided to begin our life in a new town independent of relatives and friends whose influence might serve as a distraction to our commitment to form a Christian marriage that blended our backgrounds.

We graduated from college on May 31, 1969, which was my 22nd birthday, were married on August 23rd, and began our teaching careers with the School District of Cudahy, a suburb of Milwaukee, on August 27th. Fred was hired for a fifth grade position at General Mitchell, and I was assigned a second grade at Park View. During our first three years of marriage Fred also attended graduate school at the University of Wisconsin-Milwaukee. The summer of 1972 the dual degrees of Master of Science in Educational Administration and Fatherhood were bestowed upon him. Along with both degrees came new roles and responsibilities. Fred took on an assistant principal's position and total economic responsibility for our family, as I elected to stay home with Keith during his preschool years. We bought our first house, for what a full size car costs today, when we happily discovered we were expecting our first child in November 1971.

Sylvan Drive is a cul de sac of ten houses located in the country between the two large cities of Racine and Milwaukee. Our house was a basic three bedroom ranch, but what initially attracted us to the area was the fact all the houses are on large lots, and we knew we would have great neighbors as a teacher in Fred's building already lived on the road. There were thirty playmates available when Keith grew up which provided endless hours, days, and years of fun. Keith often commented that it was the best place in the world to be brought up. A neighborhood where Summer Olympics were held, children's theater written, directed, and performed, and games for all ages preceded the annual block party. We all breathed fresh country air except when they occasionally cleaned out the pig farm a mile away, and Keith grew up on cool clear well water. Keith did not leave the area until the movers transported all of our belongings into our current house in Racine on August 16, 1990, which was the day before we moved him into the Nabor House at University of Illinois at Urbana - Champaign.

Keith energized us with his enthusiasm for life and seemingly unlimited potential, especially intellectually and athletically. He brought immeasurable joy into our home and into the lives of countless others. From little on he valued all people except kind gentle Debbie who lived across the street, who he thought was put on this earth so he could have a girl to tease. Even though Keith was a thorn in her side through their primary and elementary years by high school they had become friends, partly driven by the fact she had wheels and Keith preferred riding in a car in lieu of the "Yellow Worm" as he called the school bus.

Keith seemed to always have his priorities straight. He formed friendships with the tenacity other people collect and treasure inanimate objects. He had little interest in toys, preferring to constantly be interacting with people. A playpen was to keep his toys in, but not him. The world was for exploring. Fred devised a rubber bumper from a garden hose to place around the base of Keith's walker because he tooled around the house so fast he literally bounced off walls and doorways. He walked at eight and a half months, and at 10 months rode his stationary rocking horse with such force it actually bucked him off and knocked him out.

He always knew what he wanted and thought of creative solutions to whatever situation he found himself in, which occasionally left us shaking our heads in disbelief. At 22 months he came to the hospital with Fred to pick up his new brother Jason and me. Keith rode home in his car seat towering over his new live action toy who was peacefully sleeping in the car bed next to him. When we arrived home before Fred and I had unbuckled ourselves Keith had escaped from the constraints of his seat belt and bars, and was proudly lifting Jason up by his feet telling us he had the baby. That was the beginning of a brotherly relationship that vacillated between peanut butter and jelly and oil and water. Jason takes after his father and is a type B more relaxed personality while Keith inherited my type A active personality. Jason was a mellow child and would frequently prefer to sit and take in the action rather than be a part of it which often frustrated impatient Keith. It was not until college that their friendship solidified to the point where they became best friends.

Keith was so inquisitive his safety was always a concern so outlets were sealed, cabinets secured, and he was never far from our sight. When he was three we joined my parents and brother's family at Star Lake for a week. My brother and I learned to fish on that northern Wisconsin lake, and it was tradition grandsons learned to fish there also. We insisted Keith always wear a life jacket if he went out the cabin door. Three times that week, with six adults keeping an eye on him, he still managed to fall off the pier into the cold deep lake while observing something amazing swimming by such as a minnow, frog, or fish. He read his first 60 page book called <u>Snow</u> in kindergarten. In second grade he did his first dinosaur report which he used over and over in various forms up to and including his college years. Also in second grade he received his first shiner when I threw a ball that hit him in the eye the day of his First Communion.

Where Keith excelled academically he had little interest or ability in the fine arts, in direct contrast to his brother. When Keith was in third grade I found a piece of art work trashed in the back of his closet. We found out later it had been on display in an art show that he never told us about because one time I inadvertently thought he had drawn a cute little round pig when it really was a tiger. It made no difference to him when I tried to explain I was confused because of its curly tail and snout. He insisted I should have known it was a tiger because he used brown and yellow crayons, and I honestly believe by that mistake I took away his confidence in drawing. My only consolation is even if he had the confidence he really did have little artistic ability, so I do not think I scarred him for life. He excelled in the academics. Before Keith entered sixth grade we transferred him to Racine's Lighthouse Program at McKinley School for the gifted and talented. He had been eligible since kindergarten screening, but we really wanted to keep him in our local school because we felt it was important he learn to relate to children of all abilities, which he successfully did. However, it was at McKinley that Keith met a core of friends, from around the city, with which he explored the adventures of youth, the world of sports, and later the meaning of life.

Keith was also fortunate music was not a high school requirement. Jason received our matched recessive genes in that area for in high school he won the highest state honor for a vocal solo when he was just a freshman. In math and science our recessive genes matched up, giving Keith an understanding of contents of books where I did not even understand the title. He had a scientific mind, but the practicalities of completing an experiment were a challenge for him. He was known to blow up test tubes on a frequent basis.

Mary was his high school laboratory partner for their International Baccalaureate Science Course. Confident, caring, and capable Mary was the perfect partner for Keith. On honors night their senior year, Keith was awarded over

$20,000 dollars in scholarships and Mary over $60,000. I thought Go Mary Go, but then come back for Keith. Without Mary, Keith's science experiments at the University of Illinois had dismal results, and he credited himself for the U of I instituting a refundable user fee for scientific equipment. He never received a refund and was confident other student fees went to defray the cost of equipment lost during his failed attempts.

Keith also had a creative mind which showed up in the most surprising ways. For instance in high school he introduced us to our roots by extending our lineage beyond the factual information he found out from his grandfather. He "traced" our family history all the way back to our poor relatives in Ireland during the Great Potato Famine. Being exceptionally well written it was displayed for parent conferences which is where we first read about our heritage. We found it believable and decided until some relative actually wants to trace our lineage we'll go with Keith's version. Fortunately top grades and positive relationships with teachers came easy for Keith. After his death we received numerous letters, beginning with his first grade teacher, telling us he was the type of student that makes a lasting positive impression. Many former teachers and coaches attended his funeral where some had to stand, along with many of his friends. Friends that if we could have picked for him we would have. Friends, family, fun, and food were the F words he used in high school and beyond. We were fortunate that he never excluded us from any period of his life, and included his friends in our lives. Our dinner table was always full on lasagna and pizza nights, and the bathrooms were busy on weekends with overnight guests.

Keith's friends humorously referred to Fred and me as June and Ward Cleaver from the "Leave it to Beaver Era." Our family values may emulate the fifties, but we had successfully transposed June, Ward, and our sons into the nineties. The only traditional roles in our marriage are co-operation and commitment, everything else is up for negotiation. Fred and I are gainfully employed outside the home, Fred with the School District of South Milwaukee serving in the capacity of Principal at E. W. Luther Elementary School, and myself as the reading teacher at General Mitchell Elementary School in Cudahy. Therefore cooking, cleaning, and carrying out the garbage are everyone's responsibility. Our second family room is the laundry room where each person does their own wash. The guys do not want my help with this, because they claim I engage in chemical warfare on their clothes with my trusty bleach bottle. Fred mends, I do the taxes, we all know how to run a vacuum cleaner, lawn mower, and drive the car through an oil change station. Being outnumbered I always keep the woman's perspective front and center in terms of gender issues. Keith knew the words "that's woman's work" would guarantee a lively discussion, and we had many.

Keith did not have as much time on this earth as any of us would have wanted, but the time he did have he used wisely. From the very beginning when he decided life was too short to take such things as naps he did not waste a day. He loved more, laughed more, did more, and enjoyed more than many adults twice his age. What follows is what happened to all of us his last year of life. It is not the script any of us planned. My parents and both sets of grandparents celebrated their fiftieth wedding anniversary, and Fred's grandparents their sixty-fifth. I had envisioned a long happy life for all of us, and a future that would be bright with the addition of wives and grandchildren. Before our world was turned upside down and inside out I was busy trying to convince Keith it might be time to start thinking about finding the perfect wife, and I was already offering some suggestions. My story would have had a different ending. Now on nights when sleep is hard to come by I wonder if it is coincidence that out of our mini community of ten homes on Sylvan Drive three people contracted MS, and two have now died from the disease. I ask myself did we unknowingly raise Keith in an environment hazardous to his health?

CHAPTER TWO

St. Mary's Hospital - Madison, Wisconsin

Sept. 1, 1995: I had anticipated this September with the excitement of a child watching the Fourth of July fireworks. Our 2 sons were successfully launched on their career paths, and it was a time of financial independence for us while still enjoying their gift of presence in our lives. We had thoroughly enjoyed raising the guys, and had come through the parenting years unscathed and with a genuine friendship with our children, but were now looking forward to the financial freedom their degrees meant for us. This was the first time in five years that university tuition checks wouldn't take priority over just about any purchase. We were fortunate that both Keith and Jason completed their undergraduate work in four years due to not only determination and ability, but also the the knowledge one of the first phrases their father taught them was "four years." Keith had earned a biochemistry degree and graduated with distinction from the University of Illinois at Urbana - Champaign. Prior to his May 1994 graduation Keith was in the position of being recruited for employment. He had spent much of his spring semester flying around the country visiting chemical companies and had accepted a position with Quantum Chemical Corporation. His dad and I asked him what the deciding factor was, and he told us he always tried to get to know how the people who drove him around on company visits felt about the company. His theory was if the company drivers were happy with their employer, then it was the type of company that valued all of its employees and one he would be honored to join. Keith was always pleased with his decision to work for Quantum as a Technical Sales Representative. We were pleased with his reason.

Initially he was in a six month training program based at their corporate head-quarters in Cincinnati, Ohio which was the farthest he had ever lived from our home. But it was possible to drive there in six hours, so I handled the separation fairly successfully. In November his training was cut short when he was asked to fill a leave that was created in Philadelphia. My worry that we would not see him as often proved false, as the company flew him back to Wisconsin every other weekend. We even enjoyed a long family ski weekend with relatives at Lake Tahoe in February when Fred obtained two for one airline tickets. Actually the men skied. I liked to kid them that I could not understand how anyone in their right mind would want to pay money to acquire an aching back, burning thighs, and sore knees. While they were in ski boots I was in ice skates or hiking boots. Nights we all wore regular footwear and spent time together sharing the adventures of the day. It was our last family vacation and it was perfect.

When we came home Keith flew on to Philadelphia to complete his assignment, but returned to Cincinnati in April. Shortly after, he received his permanent territory which was Wisconsin and part of Minnesota. He moved to Madison at the beginning of June. When Keith arrived Jason had just graduated from the University of Wisconsin, and now he had also just returned to Madison to enter law school. Even though Jason was two years younger than Keith they were only a year apart in school as Jason had completed high school in three years. With both guys in Madison and the start of the Badger football season I had a lot to cheer about.

The only hint of a dark cloud in the air appeared in late August: on two specific occasions at two distinct locations, I had an unusual and strong premonition our family would soon be in crisis and that the crisis would involve Keith. Each episode I mentioned to Fred because it was something I had never experienced before. However, as uncomfortable as it felt at the time, those episodes were easy to push far back into my memory, amid the merriment of the current days.

Sept. 29th: Keith knew he wanted more education and was preparing to pursue a joint degree in business and law. His only question was whether to attend school full or part-time, as part-time would allow him to remain with Quantum. He had done well on the standardized tests for business school and was scheduled to take the law entrance exam on Saturday morning. Jason had invited him over for dinner and some last minute advice on the LSAT. When I called Jay's apartment to wish Keith good luck he seemed preoccupied, as if he were watching his forever favorite team, the Green Bay Packers, make a crucial play before he responded to my comments. After I hung up I shared with Fred how slow Keith's responses were. I did not voice concern but irritation because I perceived he was preoccupied and placating me by giving me only half of his attention.

<u>*Keith's Journal:*</u>

Sept. 29th: (Keith) This is the first day anyone said they noticed something different in my behavior. However, looking back I remember two other unusual things that happened that week. I had driven to Minneapolis on Monday, and I found myself very emotional and actually had to stop driving because of tearing. Then on Thursday when I arrived back at my apartment I was unusually tired. I slept 14 hours that night and instead of waking up refreshed was surprised what a laborious and slow process it was for me to complete my work reports. Later looking back at those reports I realized how my handwriting had changed.

Sept. 30th: A phone call from Keith woke us up shortly after six. He was calling to tell us he felt great and was off to breakfast with Jason who was then going to drive him to the exam. We wished him luck, and prayed he would do well. Since we were now awake, Fred and I decided to take an early morning bike ride to a local restaurant for breakfast. Bike riding is our hobby, in fact we rode several miles the night before Keith was born. As we have aged we've geared up with the times and now ride twenty-one speed bikes. That summer we had taken a two week bike trip with our close friends, Penny and Vern. Penny and I have been like sisters since fourth grade when we were in the same Sunday school class. She married Vern just a month before I married Fred. Fortunately our husbands also became good friends, and our families have maintained a close relationship throughout the years even though Fred and I have lived all our married life in the Racine-Milwaukee area while they remained in Madison. That summer the four of us had ridden our bikes a couple of hundred miles from inn to inn through the mountains of Vermont and along the shores of Martha's Vineyard and Nantucket Island. One night there was no room in any inn so we stayed in a Youth Hostel complete with men and women in separate dorm rooms, bunk beds, curfews, and chores. We have been biking partners for thirty years and for the last several years begin the biking season with the Chocolate Ride in May and complete the official season with the American Cancer Ride in September. Fred and I promise our sponsors if we do not complete the ride we will double their pledge but remind them it is not fair to pray for inclement weather. Now that the peak riding season had passed we were just doing some weekly recreational riding, usually from restaurant to restaurant.

When we returned home the telephone was ringing, it was Jason on the line. He was calling from his apartment with the disturbing news Keith was back and that something was terribly wrong with him. He described him as being confused, very distraught, and asking to be taken to the hospital. Trying to think clearly and sound calm, I suggested Jason take Keith to St. Mary's. When I was growing up that hospital was the one our family doctor was affiliated with, and consequently was the only one with which I was personally familiar. I then talked to Keith. I asked him if he could tell me what was wrong, and he just said he didn't know but something was, and he was really scared. I told Keith that Jay would help him get into some dry clothes and then drive him to the hospital. He seemed to understand.

Before we left I had to call our friends, Ginny and John, in Naperville, Illinois who were coming to spend the weekend with us. We have been friends for over a quarter of a century having first met when we were both newlyweds, apartment neighbors, and new to the Milwaukee area. A common need for friends began a relationship that now identifies them as part of the family. Ginny told me to keep in touch and try not to let my imagination run away with me until we knew for sure we had something to worry about. She believes Keith has had a guardian angel watching over him for a long time. When Keith was two she was baby-sitting him, and he had gone across the street with her four year old daughter to play with some other children. A short time later Keith spotted Ginny in the front yard and decided he wanted to ask her for a drink. Without looking before he crossed the street he ran directly into the path of a truck carrying a load of lumber on its roof. When the truck screeched to a halt the front bumper was inches from Keith, and the load of lumber had flown over him and was strewn all over the road behind him. Keith was literally standing between two forces that could have easily killed him. Now with the ringing of the telephone I was identifying with the panic she felt hearing those squealing tires and brakes.

The drive from Racine to Madison seemed unbearably long because of anxiety, road construction, and a car fire that had temporarily shut down all west lanes of the freeway. We had a car phone so were able to keep abreast with what was happening to Keith which was primarily diagnostic testing. By the time we finally arrived, Keith was resting comfortably. I will never forget the emergency room doctor who told us he had run a blood test and could assure us **100%** nothing was physically wrong with Keith. That was to be the first of many doctors wearing white coats accessorized with black stethoscopes who would deliver diagnoses to us. I have little recollection of the medical messengers, but I clearly remember the messages. I focus on personalities instead of looks. When my husband shaved off the mustache he had worn for 15 years I never realized it until Jason's girlfriend, Carrie, pointed it out to me when she saw him that night. When kidded about it I said that it just confirmed I didn't marry Fred for his good looks, but his winning personality. This doctor's personality was one of genuine confidence and he proudly prefaced his remarks by informing us of his title within the hospital. He felt Keith was on stress overload compounded by a possible drug reaction to his allergy medicine and medication he had taken for what he thought was a migraine headache. TALK ABOUT JUSTIFICATION FOR A SECOND OPINION! Shortly after, Keith was released, Fred and I spent the night with him. I was so relieved nothing was seriously wrong I didn't worry about the fact he still seemed somewhat dazed and a little confused. Whatever it was we were told it was going to pass. Fred referred to it as waiting for him to return from "La La Land."

Sept. 30th: (Keith) When I arrived at the LSAT I began filling out the personal identification portion of the exam. I had spent over 200 hours preparing for this test and felt confident. I do not get nervous in exams and on numerous occasions during my undergraduate work counted on exams to counteract the hours I spent on the basketball court instead of keeping up with daily work. My practice scores had given me the confidence I needed to feel I would do well. However, once in the exam I realized the person giving the instructions had moved onto a different section and I had no memory of what had just happened. I found myself hurrying to catch up, but my thought process was slowing down more and more. I began the exam, but couldn't remember anything I read and found myself reading and rereading with little or no comprehension. When the break came I turned in my test, walked out in the pouring rain, and somehow made it back to my brother's apartment although I have no recollection of how I got there. When I got there I couldn't release my wallet from one hand or my keys from the other. Realizing something was terribly wrong I asked Jason to take me to the hospital. I remember very little after that until I awoke and found Mom and Dad in the room with me. When the doctor came back with his diagnosis I knew he was wrong, but wanted to believe that perhaps I really would be okay in a few hours. Back at my apartment I still felt like I was in a fog and began to experience some aphasia. For instance when I walked into my kitchen I recognized all my appliances but could not recall the name for the stove. I remembered it was something to cook food on. I was also starting to use my left hand instead of my right. Mom asked why I closed the car door with my left hand and I had no idea.

Oct. 1st: In the morning Keith appeared better, and we felt comfortable leaving him alone while we went to church. My ceaseless prayers, that were more like pleas, on the way to Madison had been answered, and I wanted to formally thank God. Later Jason came over, and the four of us went to the Olive Garden for lunch. Jason planned to spend the remainder of the day and night with Keith, so Fred and I left for Racine. We felt if it was stress overload the last thing he needed was Mother smother, and by leaving we'd be conveying the message we thought he would be fine, just as the doctor said.

On our drive home the radio played the old song "Turn Turn Turn" by the Byrds with the line "There is a Time for Every Season Under Heaven." It was then I remembered the premonitions I had in August, and told Fred that I was suddenly afraid this was our time for trouble. Fred was quite confident the doctor was right and Keith would be fine, but that night Jason called to say Keith was confused again. The emergency room doctor was so positive nothing was seriously wrong with Keith he didn't even give us the name of a doctor to reach in case Keith experienced any additional problems, so I called the emergency room. The nurse gave no indication I should be alarmed since I told her the doctor was 100% sure nothing was physically wrong with Keith, but suggested if symptoms continued it would be wise to have him reevaluated, and I was given the name of a neurologist to contact Monday morning.

Oct. 1st: (Keith) I woke up more alert but still had a headache. After Mom and Dad left Jason and I went to Kinko's to make copies of the paperwork I needed to officially cancel my LSAT scores and to register for the next exam. While there I became very confused and upset because I could not remember how to use the copier. Jason calmed me down, suggested we come back later, and on the way back to my apartment he stopped at the video store to pick up a couple of no brainers. During the movies he called Mom and Dad. I hated to worry them.

Oct. 2nd: Jason took Keith to the neurologist. Shortly after lunch Fred called me at school to tell me Keith was being admitted to the hospital for observation. We decided I would leave school immediately and go to Madison just in case there were any unforeseen problems. We were still operating under the 100% guarantee there was nothing physically wrong with Keith. I left school and 10 minutes after my arrival at the hospital Keith was told by the woman neurologist who had admitted him he had two brain masses. I quickly informed the doctor she was mistaken because on Saturday we were given a 100% guarantee there was nothing physically wrong. She told us that doctor was wrong because an MRI revealed two masses. The official report described them as a massive cystic structure in the left rolandic area and a separate lesion in the posterior aspect of the corpus callosum.

Suddenly I felt like all the air was being sucked out of the room. It was as if I were in an echo chamber and those fateful words just kept bouncing around my brain without being absorbed. It couldn't be. Keith was the perfect candidate for the cover of the magazine <u>Men's Health</u>. He was always concerned about eating right and getting plenty of exercise. Fit, trim, and good-looking, he was the picture of health and worked constantly to maintain that image. He felt a day without significant physical activity was a day wasted. Tennis, running, golf, hiking, skiing, and especially basketball were his advocations. To demonstrate just how important basketball was to Keith, the following story should suffice. During the spring semester of his senior year he was enrolled in a course where the professor recorded attendance. Due to a number of absences because of job interviews he felt compelled to be in class when on campus. However, on one particularly warm early spring day while sitting in class by an open window, he thought he could hear the basketball hoop calling his name. Therefore, following attendance, when the instructor turned his back to unlock the computer cabinet Keith dove out the window to the astonishment of those sitting around him. He landed in the bushes several feet below, climbed out, and according to eye witnesses took off running towards his beloved hoop. Once he graduated he continued to play B-ball as he called it, and it had only been six weeks since his team had won the 3-on-3 Hoop It Up Basketball Tournament for their division in Milwaukee. He had also just returned from a strenuous backpacking trip in the Rocky Mountains. Keith was perpetual motion and energized his body with only the right foods. Jason always joked, "Keith treats his body like a temple, and I treat mine like an amusement park." I remember thinking, I have to call Fred, I have to get some air, I have to wake up from this nightmare.

Within minutes after the doctor left a nurse came to pad Keith's bed because a cat-scan had also indicated the possibility of seizure activity. Then a neurosurgeon arrived. His opening comment was "This hasn't been a very good day for you." He was wrong. A not-very-good day is when I lock the keys in my car with the engine running, a three hour dental appointment, or the sewer backing up in the basement. This was the WORST day of my life, and it didn't compare to a bad day. After he finished terrorizing me with the facts, I escaped from the hospital by fleeing to Keith's apartment to gather his personal items and to notify his boss, our family, and friends who began numerous and important prayer chains. What is unsettling is I must have been in a partial state of shock as I have absolutely no recollection of driving to or from Keith's apartment.

While I was gone Keith called his Uncle Fred in Kansas City who is my only sibling. There is a seven year age difference between us due to World War II, and because of such an age gap, we never interacted very much until I grew up and married my Fred. By the time Keith and Jason were born my brother already had three sons. Shortly after my boys came along, Fred and Linda had Scott and Adam making a total of seven guys available for the many physical activities they engaged in. Actually it was eight because my brother always went out to play with them, so Keith felt particularly close to him. Uncle Fred was his basketball, softball, football, tennis, ping-pong, pool, golf, jogging, swimming, skiing, and backpacking partner.

Keith also called Phil, his fraternity brother and closest college friend. They met when Keith was a sophomore and Phil was a freshman. Phil was Keith's fraternity "little brother." They became immediate friends sharing a passion for wholesome fun and sports. They roomed together for three of the four years Keith lived at the Nabor House. Although his relationship with Phil was special, Keith truly became like a brother to many of the men of Nabor House Agricultural Fraternity. Keith's fraternity nickname was Cheese and it was one of his goals to make all his "brothers" Packer Cheeseheads. Nabor House is an independent fraternity that emulates the values Keith was raised with such as encouraging regular church attendance. The house promotes education by not allowing alcoholic beverages inside the house and rewards the 50% of the fraternity brothers with the highest grade points with steak at the semi-annual steak and bean dinner. Only once Keith ate beans, the semester his grandfather died. Keith stood up with Phil when he married Carissa and they now had a little daughter named Briana whom we all adored. The three of them had recently spent the weekend with us when Phil and Keith participated in the Hoop It Up Tournament.

Oct. 2nd: (Keith) I was somewhat relieved to realize that I was not going crazy and actually something was physically wrong with me. After the neurologist broke the news, she sent the neurosurgeon to explain the two possible procedures for the brain biopsy. When the neurosurgeon finished talking about the procedure he was recommending, I asked Mom and Jason to leave the room. I then asked the doctor the worst case scenario and was told death was imminent without surgery. I was told the masses could either be tumors or a brain infection. Being a pro-active person I elected to have the brain biopsy done the next day under local anesthesia. I was glad Jason stayed the night as we spent most of the time talking, at one point, becoming so loud impersonating the "Jerky Boys," a nurse came in to see if we were okay. No, I was not okay, but I knew one thing and that was I didn't want to die. My life was just beginning and whatever this was I intended to fight it.

Oct. 3rd. Most people remember this day as the day the O.J. Simpson criminal verdict came back. For me it was the day God reminded me who is in control of life, and it is not a jury of peers. Fred and I had spent the night in Jason's apartment which was within walking distance to the hospital. When Fred awoke, from a couple of restless hours of sleep, he shared he did not want to face this day and I agreed with him. At the hospital we met my brother, Linda, and Adam who had flown in from Kansas City on a red-eye flight. Soon Mom, her pastor, and Fred's dad and step-mother joined us. We also knew Phil, Carissa, and numerous fraternity brothers were en route. Our long-time friends Penny and Vern became constants at the hospital, and they all enveloped us that day with their physical, emotional, and spiritual support. Countless others had been notified and were holding us up in prayer. The surgeon sent a nurse to talk to us that he had successfully performed brain surgery on using local anesthesia. Her words were comforting and reassuring that Keith was literally in good hands. I had also talked to other staff members about the surgeon and was told that even if Keith had gone to another hospital in Madison most likely he would have been transferred to St. Mary's because this doctor was considered the expert for this surgical procedure. He was one of very few in the state who was trained to perform this type of operation under local anesthetic. We were told for the patient the advantage of local anesthetic was it greatly reduces the risk of loss of function during the procedure. Using probes and Keith's verbal responses they planned to literally map the route into Keith's brain so as to avoid any area that controls motor function. We had our first look at the affected area as shown on the MRI, and it was massive.

I felt events were going too fast and we were spiraling out of control, but Keith was 23 and we wanted him to make his own decisions. Keith had always done things quickly, waiting was not part of his lifestyle. Yet, I had not built a trust relationship with this hospital as we were getting a lot of varying information. The first doctor had told us nothing was physically wrong with Keith, the second said because of the size of the mass most likely it was a slow growing tumor that had been growing for at least two years, while the surgeon suggested it could be an infection. So I asked Jason if he thought it would be okay if I called Carrie's father who is a doctor and ask him if we should encourage Keith to seek another opinion at another medical facility. Both Carrie and Jason said her dad would be glad to help in anyway he could. When I reached him he assured me the suggested procedure was appropriate because it would be impossible to begin any treatment plan without knowing exactly what the problem was. This doctor I trusted.

Surgery was scheduled for three o'clock and the hours went quickly without much time to absorb this horrific turn of events in our lives. We shared, laughed, cried, prayed, and somehow found the strength to stay with Keith through all the medical procedures before he left for surgery. My last words to him at the elevator were "Feel His power Keith, feel His power."

When Keith went to surgery, Fred and I went to the chapel. I was always amazed how waiting rooms are always full with people watching television, and how empty the chapels are. I really had no idea what to say to God except to acknowledge I believed Keith was indeed a gift and I knew God was aware no son could be loved more. I felt he belonged to both of us, and therefore we both needed to help him. I did not make any promises if He would heal Keith nor any threats if He wouldn't. I just kept praying we would become aware of His presence. Like doubting Thomas, I needed to somehow be able to feel His power. At 5:15 p.m. an indescribable peace simultaneously came over my husband and me. It was a feeling we have never felt before or since, yet the warmth and intensity of that experience has carried us through to this very day.

My brother came shortly after to tell us the surgeon wanted to speak with us up in the Intensive Care Unit. Always be suspicious if a doctor tells you to sit down. Actually he ordered me to sit. When I walked in he suggested I sit down. I told him I was fine, and he repeated his suggestion to sit. When I hesitated he sat down and patted the space next to him insisting I join him. Once I was seated he told us the mass looked like something he had never seen before and the initial reports indicated they were abnormal cells but not cancer cells. The reason he had me sit was the devastating news which was to follow, Keith had lost mobility on his right side. The official medical report said:

> The frozen section diagnosis was indeterminate; described the tissue as abnormal containing macrophages, lymphocytes, and inflammatory cells, but a definite diagnosis could not be identified. During the procedure, the patient became weak on his right side which was difficult to explain given the distance that we were away from his motor cortex as mapped out and his speech remained intact. We gave him some extra Decadron during the procedure. We had adequate tissue for sampling, and then we elected to back out and to see if his weakness would improve.

I asked him why Keith lost movement and he had no idea. At which point he began drawing us a diagram detailing how, with Keith's verbal guidance, he had mapped out the area where the motor section was and he was far from the area when Keith lost movement. He said in layman's terms he was a mile away from the critical area. While the doctor delivered that somber message the recovery room called and said Keith had begun to move his right side. Immediately a cheer erupted from the numerous family members and friends who were in the room with us.

Within a few hours Keith was brought to the Intensive Care Unit flashing a thumbs up with his left hand. His nurse allowed everyone the opportunity to briefly see him in groups of two. Several shared that Keith told them he had a revelation that he would be fine. When Fred and I saw him he told us how good it was to see us and how much he loved us.

That night, after everyone left the hospital feeling confident the worst was behind, Fred and I went to get a cup of hot chocolate. When we returned, which was now 11 o'clock, Penny had just arrived back at the hospital and was standing by the nurse who conveyed Keith had again stopped moving, and they were calling the surgical team back to the hospital. Penny literally upheld me and then slept on the floor beside us as we kept vigil through the long night. Before the team arrived, Keith began moving again. It was now about midnight and the thought occurred to me no one goes to visit people at a hospital at 11:00 at night. I began to realize events were happening that just could not be coincidence; my friend's late night presence, the earlier premonitions followed by the indescribable sense of peace Fred and I felt when Keith was in surgery, and the revelation Keith spoke of. But I was too physically and emotionally exhausted to invest any energy into trying to figure it all out.

Oct. 3rd: (Keith) So much happened so quickly I really didn't have time to absorb the impact of this day until an hour before surgery when I broke down and told my parents I was too young to die. Mom told me to put my trust in God and just to try and "Feel His power." That was also the last thing I remember her telling me before the elevator door closed. I learned the true meaning of physical pain and it is brain shots. Nothing has ever come close to the searing pain of those five shots. I tell people you could break all my fingers at once and the pain would be less than what I felt with each of those shots. I couldn't believe my family stayed with me while they were administered, but I like to tease my Mom that she didn't watch so being there didn't count. The surgery itself was not an unpleasant experience. I was alert, responsive, and very aware of my surroundings. Everything was in the realm of real until somewhere near the end when I experienced a profound revelation. I can't describe it except to say it was a warmth that enveloped my entire being, and I was given the knowledge that I would be fine, but no timeline was given. This assurance was so powerful I will never doubt or deny what I experienced. Therefore I wasn't afraid when I couldn't move nor surprised when I could. It was good to give my fraternity brothers and family a thumbs up when I returned to the ICU. I told them about the revelation which I believe is the first time I ever initiated a conversation about a religious experience. Later I remember the nurse telling my parents I had stopped moving, but I knew I could move it was just exhausting and really hard work. It took all my effort to muster the strength to move, so that I wouldn't have to go through anymore tests. Being in ICU was difficult in the sense rest was next to impossible as it seemed someone was always asking me to do something. Finally, when they asked me to urinate I was so proud I could comprehend and comply I filled the entire container and had them keep it on the shelf as my trophy. The only way they could remove it was if they would let me return to my room on the neurological floor. It worked because a few hours later I was moved out of ICU without my trophy.

Oct. 4th: Fred and I told Keith about the sense of peace we had experienced during his surgery. The previous night was the first time he spoke with such conviction about the personal presence of God in his life. Keith attended church, and in the past we had countless hours of religious discussions, but he always kidded about placing his hopes for salvation on the idea God might grade on a curve and he would be able to slip in. He was intrigued with our experience and later, through communication with his surgical nurse, we discovered we had all independently yet simultaneously experienced the sense of God's presence at exactly the same time: 5:15p.m. The current problem was revelation and reality were antonyms as Keith was getting worse. It was the first, but not the last time I felt God was contradicting Himself.

Oct. 5th: This was one of our lowest days. Keith had basically lost his speech and had very little movement. The only thing that kept me going was the incredible amount of support we were receiving. We were constantly surrounded by family and friends. Keith's room had over 20 flower arrangements ranging from dozens of fragrant roses to peace plants in full bloom and over three dozen brightly colored balloons floating overhead conveying messages of cheer. Literally everywhere I turned I was reminded we were not going through this alone.

That day the surgeon, who was originally from Canada, told me the only diagnosis that made any sense to him was a rare form of Multiple Sclerosis he became aware of while attending a conference in Canada. He explained because Saint Mary's was unable to come up with a definitive diagnosis the lab slides were now going to be sent to the Mayo Clinic for further study. He concluded his remarks with the generalization that no matter what the final diagnosis was we had a long road ahead of us. Those ended up to be very prophetic words. Knowing what I heard was not positive news I never discussed what he said with anyone except Fred and Jason.

Keith needed help with everything, and you could tell in his eyes just how sad he was. Keith was known for his contagious laugh, wonderful sense of humor, and the perpetual sparkle in his eyes…that sparkle never completely returned. We knew that his thought process was in place, but he just couldn't find the words to effectively communicate with us. We knew when we were wrong in our guesses, which was most of the time, because he could say "NO!" I can remember Keith trying to say he wanted cereal and the closest he could get was to say "Tony Tiger" when he meant Frosted Flakes. Similarly, we quickly realized that "lemon-lime taste" meant he wanted soda.

At one point Fred and I left Keith with family members and went to the cafeteria to share our thoughts. We felt we had to make some long term care and work decisions. Initially we were told Keith would only be in the hospital three or four days. Now it was apparent we were far from recovery and going the wrong direction. Knowing the seriousness of the decisions we were facing I was extremely irritated with the server at the cafeteria who was impatiently waiting for me to decide if I wanted rice or potatoes. The routines of life suddenly seemed absurd to me, nothing was normal or routine in our lives and I wondered if it ever would be again. After much discussion we decided I would take a family medical leave, but if Keith did not significantly improve we would need some outside support with his care.

Another major concern was Jason who was considering dropping out of law school. He had basically missed a week of classes and didn't know if he could handle the stress of being a first year law student and his constant desire to be with his brother, his best friend. Later that night we decided to leave Keith alone for an hour to help Jason decern his decision. From the beginning Fred and I were very cognizant of the fact we had two sons we loved and did not want two lives destroyed. Outside the door, standing in the pouring rain, was another good friend trying to get in. There must be 20 ways into the hospital, and I do not believe it was coincidence a friend was waiting at that particular locked door. We had begun to refer to these experiences as "God sightings." Our friend brought us good cheer, and his father, who is a minister, called later to assure us you walk though the valley of the shadow of death, you don't stay there.

Oct. 6th: Finally events were taking a major turn for the better so my brother Fred, Linda, and Adam felt comfortable leaving, but my husband's family readily took their place. Fred is the oldest of five children. He has three married sisters, Barb, Marlene, and Diane. His brother Tom now owns the dairy farm where they all grew up. Tom and Diane were Keith's godparents. Each family was keeping in close contact with us and taking turns making the trip from the Fond du Lac area to Madison.

Keith's speech had also begun to return. He could tell us when he needed to use the bathroom, and with the assistance of two nurses he took his first halting steps as that day he refused to urinate except in the bathroom. Because he wanted the room kept dark, quiet, and cold our relatives and friends literally took over the waiting room and individually took turns sitting with Keith. Even staff members began referring to Keith's room as "The Cave."

In many ways it was good to see him reclaim control of his environment, but in some ways it was scary because he really wasn't Keith as we knew him. For instance Keith never used bad language around me and was always extremely courteous to people. Among the books he owned was <u>Don't Slurp Your Soup in Public.</u> Manners were important to Keith. Therefore it was disconcerting when I heard him tell a nurse, "You better be pregnant, otherwise you are really fat." Fortunately, she was pregnant. She told me not to feel embarrassed because many people who have brain disfunction lose their speech inhibitions temporarily. Later in the day my mom was sitting next to him when he asked her, "What's that noise?" She replied the only sound was her breathing, and he told her to stop so he could sleep.

Following that episode I went with Mom to the cafeteria to get something to eat. I was eating bananas and toast because I had no appetite. On her tray was a layered dessert of pastry, creams, and fruits representing a month's total of the recommended daily amount of fat grams and something she normally would never have eaten as she is very calorie conscious. I inquired if she really intended to eat that decadence of delight. She answered in the affirmative, and I acknowledged desserts spelled backwards is stressed, which we certainly all were. She also reminded me that Keith only ate health foods, and she wasn't impressed with the results she was seeing. I had to agree with her.

Jason had talked to the Dean of the Law School who encouraged him to try and stay in school. He supported Jason's personal need to be with Keith, and said he would authorize a drop at a later date as he did not want Jason's decision driven by the scheduled drop date. By choice, Jason was now in the uncomfortable position of sitting at a school desk all day and sleeping in a recliner at the hospital all night.

Oct. 6th: (Keith) Losing one's speech is horrible. Just trying to communicate the basics like having to go to the bathroom became an exhausting and frustrating task. I knew exactly what I wanted to say, but the words just would not surface. Now improvements are happening so rapidly I look forward to waking up from naps. Each time I wake I can do more. The doctors are pretty confident what I have is a rare form of MS. It presents itself like a stroke, and usually one can expect a full recovery without any further episodes. When sharing that diagnosis the surgeon told me at the time of surgery he was 90% sure he was operating on a brain tumor with a short life expectancy. I just know I am going to be fine. The only drugs I am receiving are a steroid called Decadron for inflammation and Dilantin as a precaution so I do not experience a seizure both of which they began before surgery. Jason told me he is thinking about dropping out of school, but I told him I am going to get better and will go on with my life so I think he should stay in school. I sure hope he does.

Oct. 8th: Keith's movements had accelerated to the point that Jason had converted Keith's practice walks into a synchronized walking routine to entertain the nursing staff. They would circle around the nurses station linked arm in arm doing a left, right, kick step. Wanting a more formal assessment of Keith's progress, his neurologist had requested an evaluation of his current level of functioning by a doctor from Meriter Hospital. That particular hospital has a reputation for its outstanding rehabilitation department and is just down the street from St. Mary's. A physician had visited and at the conclusion of the exam recommended Keith transfer to Meriter for one or two weeks of intense rehabilitation therapy. This doctor told us that following brain trauma most healing occurs within the first four weeks. Therefore time was of essence and it was important for Keith to receive more hours of therapy than was currently possible at St. Mary's. Keith understood what was shared and agreed to the transfer.

With such dramatic improvement we felt Fred could leave and return to work. Before leaving the area he stopped at my mom's to pick up our dog. It was while retrieving Sam, Fred decided he felt too uncomfortable going home and elected to stay one more night. At the hospital Fred and I often wished we could get away, but when we did leave we worried until we returned. We were currently living a life where peace, contentment, and happiness were illusions and nowhere to be found; which was in direct contrast to our previous life of peace, contentment, and happiness.

Jason slept at the hospital with Keith, and I met Fred at Keith's apartment. On that cool autumn night, huddled together on his deck under a harvest moon, we reflected on the unbelievable events of the past week. Prior to September 30th many people felt we had the luck of the Irish, but now certainly no one was calling us the luckiest family they knew. Fortunately they were still calling, visiting, praying, and supporting us in ways that were making a difference in our ability to cope. Fred and I reconfirmed our love for each other and promised with the help of God, our family, and friends to continue to be there for each other and our sons regardless of what the future held.

Oct. 9th: I wired a dozen long stem red roses to Fred at work as a symbol of my love and appreciation for the strength with which he held us all together since that alarming phone call from Jason. We all kid Fred about his need for organization and the importance of calendars in his life, but we all relied on his clarity of thought and detailed notes as we worked our way through the medical jargon and implications of the numerous doctor patient bedside conversations. Once home Fred engaged in two more difficult dialogues. Our family had the privilege of hosting two terrific foreign exchange students, Joe and Morgana. Both of them lived with us during their senior year of high school. Joe is from Spain, and he stayed with us 14 years ago. We have always kept in touch, and were disappointed we were unable to attend his March of '94' wedding due to our school calendars. However, Joe and Nuria elected to spend part of their honeymoon with us. Our second student Morgana from Curitiba, Brazil was living with us at the time, and I found it amazing they got to meet each other. As the guys also came home from their respective universities that spring weekend we literally had all our children together for the first and last time.

Keith had already purchased his plane ticket to spend the holidays in Brazil with Morgana. All three of them were saddened by the unexpected news, but hopeful Keith would continue to improve.

Oct. 10th: That morning I was inattentively walking towards Keith's room when I became an observer in a real life and death drama. A patient on a gurney coded in front of me, not behind me, or beside me, but directly in front of me. From seemingly out of nowhere medical staff arrived and I was literally trapped in the action. I stood there frozen in absolute shock and amazement thinking I was on a television set. After a blur of activity the woman began breathing again and was rushed off. Within seconds the corridor was clear, and it was hard to comprehend that what I had witnessed was not acting. I subconsciously expected someone to step forward and say, "That's a wrap." I admire people who can react calmly regardless of the situation, but I am not one of them. While they all returned to their normal duties I was hyperventilating in Keith's room trying to describe what had just transpired in the hall. Later in the day I had another surprise, but this one was pleasant. I found a fraternity brother in Keith's bed and Keith taking a shower. Keith was improving at a rapid rate. The guys had ordered a pizza, and Keith used his right hand to eat. I was actually relaxed and enjoyed the light heartedness of their conversation thinking I had come a long way in my ability to function within a hospital setting. The doctors had told Keith even though he had the most cheerful room in the hospital, thanks to the generosity of people who wanted to tangibly show their support, he still had to leave in the morning. He would leave without a final pathology report, but that night it appeared our prayers were now being answered and Keith would be fine.

CHAPTER THREE

Meriter Hospital - Madison, WI

Oct. 11th: Keith was up and anxious to be discharged when I arrived at the hospital. While Keith was complaining to his nurse about having to follow hospital policy and ride out in a wheelchair, my friend Penny and I loaded her van and my car with all the cards, gifts, flowers, and balloons he had received. A little while later as Keith was being reluctantly wheeled down the hall, we passed the surgeon who 10 days ago looked me in the eye and said the advantage of local anesthesia was the dramatically reduced risk of losing function from the procedure. This morning he avoided eye contact with me. I never felt he was responsible for what happened to Keith, but I would have appreciated eye contact. He did speak to Keith, and perhaps there were no words for us to exchange. The day of Keith's surgery I told him I was turning over to him the best I had to offer which was one of my children, and all I asked of him was his best, which I believe he gave us. Unfortunately, for all of us, best was not good enough as Keith was being transferred to another hospital instead of his home. Keith was transported by hospital van to Meriter's Physical Medicine and Rehabilitation Inpatient Unit to "maximize his functional recovery from his left hemisphere brain lesion."

Penny and I went ahead to decorate his new environment, which was an extremely large room with four beds that he shared with a teenager recovering from a coma precipitated by a motorcycle accident several months earlier. When Keith arrived I witnessed his determination. The admitting nurse wanted to take Keith on a tour of the floor and intended to put a gait belt on him. The belt goes around a patient's waist and allows the medical staff some leverage with which to support the person. No way was Keith going to wear one. He made it very clear that he was quite capable of moving independently and did not want, nor would accept, any assistance. It was encouraging to see his confidence rebound. Keith won and never wore a belt during his stay at Meriter as his mobility and balance continued to improve.

Oct. 12th: The first two days were used for assessment which, from my perspective, amounted to a deficit demonstration. Initially, the process irritated me. When Keith's vocabulary was evaluated, it was obvious to me when he reached his level of functioning, but the speech therapist continued to give him vocabulary list after vocabulary list. Keith was pronouncing words fine, but was being evaluated by the speech therapist because he was having trouble with word retrieval. Keith was asked to respond to a set sequence of words. Only after he missed a specific number of words in succession would the assessment stop. When Keith was near his current vocabulary level he would consistently miss about seven or eight words in a row then answer one correctly and proceed to miss another seven or eight. It was obvious he was aware he was getting far more wrong than right, and I did not feel he needed to know just how high the mountain was to recovery. Finally I could not contain myself and asked her to please stop. She said the test would not be valid. I wanted to choke her.

As a reading specialist, I assess children all the time and believe there is a way to do it that eliminates frustration. When I evaluate children it isn't important finding out if they are reading at a second grade first month or second month of reading if continuing the assessment causes them anxiety. Once I know the range of their ability I have a starting point. It was obvious that Keith's vocabulary was around the 12th grade, and I did not care about having valid test results if it meant devaluing Keith, my son, who graduated with honors, had a vocabulary that placed him in the 99% on standardized tests, and until the end of September was managing millions of dollars of accounts.

When we left, I was extremely upset and frustrated. The craziness of it all was Keith handled it fine and said he thought it would be better if I didn't go to speech with him anymore. On the first day of being his support person I got myself fired. He never allowed me back in the speech room. I made sure I was quiet in occupational and physical therapy so to always be invited to return.

At Meriter the staff prefers to have someone attend the therapies with the patient. Keith's program was set up so he would have five hours of therapy each day, which was a significant amount of time. Every morning and afternoon he would meet with his physical and occupational therapists. Keith viewed those women as his personal trainers, and he enjoyed getting a specific exercise routine established. Being used to working out he was familiar with the different weights and most of the exercises. The problem was he always wanted to take each exercise to the next level of difficulty and push himself. If they suggested five pound ankle weights he'd convince them seven was better. He constantly tried to do more and so was always ready for a nap during his two hour break after lunch.

Each day I would use his down time to go for long reflective walks. Often I would try to reconstruct and clarify in my own mind those previous premonitions and the sense of God's presence Fred and I experienced the day of Keith's surgery. Both premonitions occurred in late August when I was with Fred. The first was on a Saturday morning when we were returning from grocery shopping. We were less than a half mile from our home when I suddenly had this definite feeling that something bad was about to happen to Keith. It came out of nowhere as we were not talking about Keith, and yet it was unsettling in its intensity. I shared with Fred what had just occurred by describing it as a really weird thought.

After I told him, I felt better, and we both tried to dismiss it from our minds because we knew Keith was fine. He had just recently returned from a strenuous backpacking trip in the Rocky Mountains with his Uncle Fred and cousins Jeff, Scott, and Adam which he thoroughly enjoyed. Even though it was his first trip, and he went with experienced hikers, he had absolutely no trouble keeping up with them. In fact Jeff and Keith were often in the lead. Visualizing him hiking left little room for concern.

The second premonition occurred sometime later when Fred and I were taking one of our regular evening walks through our subdivision. As clearly as I remember the feeling I know the exact location where it happened. We were just approaching the common area which includes a pond within a park-like setting. That time when I told Fred I probed the experience a little further and said it felt like someone was sending me a barely audible distress signal warning me significant trouble was ahead involving Keith. We then admitted serious trouble had never really infiltrated our nucleus of four, but if it did we would need to face it with courage and faith. After that I never really thought about those episodes again as I am not the type of person that even reads horoscopes let alone pretends to have any advance knowledge of what the future holds.

However, two months later in the current context of my life, those premonitions took on new meaning. Were we indeed forewarned, and if so I wondered why? Then I also pondered over what Fred and I experienced in the chapel the day of Keith's surgery. I definitely had prayed for a sense of God's presence, and now the ever present question in my mind was, did He respond?

I believe the answer is yes. Fred and I were sitting quietly with our own thoughts when a warmth enveloped me. The best description I can give is to imagine being outside on a cool cloudy day when suddenly the sun breaks through the clouds and for a brief time you feel the warmth of those rays permeate your entire body. I was totally immersed in that kind of warmth and sense of well being. At the time I was simultaneously comfortable and uncomfortable with what was happening, so I interrupted the silence to ask Fred if he was experiencing anything unusual without using any prompts or descriptors as to what I was feeling. He said he felt different and there was a sense of total peace overtaking him. Then it passed. Both of us consider ourselves rational human beings so even though what happened appeared to be irrational the reality was we did experience a peace that defies human explanation or description. The question I kept dealing with on those soul searching afternoon walks was if indeed this was a "God sighting" why had God chosen us to manifest his presence?

Never exactly sure what direction I would go when I walked out the front door of Meriter Hospital I always knew I would end up back in the chapel at St. Mary's hoping and praying God would again meet me there in a very tangible way, but it never happened. Fall colors had arrived in Madison and there was a beauty that was in direct contrast to the storm of confusion and frustration that was building inside of me.

Walking forward under the bright blue autumn sky surrounded by a profusion of color, I constantly had to tell the devil of doubts to get behind me. Outwardly I was appearing to hold it together, but inwardly I was feeling overwhelmed. Besides struggling with the whole spiritual issue, I found being in a rehabilitation setting hard. Seeing the devastation that accidents cause on lives almost made me physically sick. Some patients were there because they were the innocent victims of a car accident which made the world suddenly seem like a dangerous place where even crossing the street became risky. Aware others were there because of lapses of judgment such as diving into shallow water without checking the depth, or riding a motorcycle without a helmet on a hot day sat uncomfortably with me. I felt they were sentenced to unreasonably cruel and permanent punishment for the crime of giving into the impulses of youth. Other patients were there because of eating, smoking, or lifestyle habits. I could not figure out why Keith was there. Yes, he exposed himself to risks, for example skiing at breakneck speeds the advanced trails at Squaw Valley, but he was not in a rehabilitation setting because of an injury. Nor was he there because of substance abuse. He always felt blessed he had such a strong healthy body and never took it for granted. The best I could come up with was an uncomfortable sense that God was demonstrating through us the folly of having total confidence in one's own ability to control one's destiny.

Following Keith's naps afternoons were spent in therapies we both enjoyed. Usually we would either be in Meriter's full size gym or outside. The gym was located on the top floor of the hospital and was completely surrounded by glass which offered a breathtaking panoramic view of the city. In the gym I would do laps on the circular track while Keith worked out on the equipment in the center. Daily exercise was important for both of us. About the time we were done Jason would arrive, and most nights friends and or relatives would also join us for an evening of visiting and playing board games. Surprisingly time passed quickly.

Oct. 12th: (Keith) Arriving at Meriter was like being given a second chance at life. Outside the dining area is a deck that I enjoy sitting out on just thinking how lucky I am to be alive. God has given me a second chance, and I'm not about to waste it. I look forward to the daily visits from my relatives and friends. At St. Mary's my phone was disconnected because I needed the rest, and I did not have the language skills to communicate. Here, I answer calls and spend time after visiting hours making them. My memory has returned to the point where I can recall my parents calling card number so I haven't tried to remember my own. Relatives are not allowed overnight and that's good as it gives me a chance to practice regaining my independence. Walking down the hall to shower and shave is wonderful. Heading out to the nurses station to joke with the staff is fun. Each therapy session represents a new opportunity to regain some of my previous function which is tiring but extremely satisfying. Walking to Hardee's with my physical therapist was great. It didn't bother me in the least I had absolutely no sense of direction because that has always been a problem. Getting back in a gym, lifting weights, actually jogging

Oct. 15th: To an outsider it would have appeared we were just enjoying a typical October weekend in Wisconsin. Fred had driven in Wednesday night, but I still missed him and was relieved and pleased he was back. He keeps our family on an even keel while I am more emotional and over-reactive. His physical presence literally has a calming effect on me. Keith had been allowed to return to his apartment Saturday and Sunday on day passes. It was exciting, standing on his third floor deck, welcoming him home knowing he would have no trouble navigating the steps to greet those waiting for him. His apartment was already filled with the sounds of laughter created by the numerous family members, friends, and fraternity brothers gathered to celebrate his arrival with him. With ideal weather Keith's apartment was large enough to handle the overflow crowd as his deck became party center. There was the aroma of almost constant grilling of dozens of brats and hamburgers which Keith had gone shopping for with his dad. The two of them frequently experienced kitchen calamities, but they were a dynamic duo on the grill. On Sunday, while Fred manned the Weber, Keith went on a two mile walk with Jason, my brother, and his cousin Adam. Later when I caught a glimpse of them returning through the park the scene was so natural even I was amazed how far Keith had come in such a short time. So it surprised me when my brother and I were eating lunch I caught myself saying I still was not sure this was over. He chided me as I have always been the family optimist, and he could not fathom how I could have any doubts that Keith wasn't on the road to a quick and complete recovery. I couldn't either, but I did.

Oct. 16th: When Fred called I told him Keith was not as good as he had been Sunday. Fred assured me he probably was just tired from all the activity. In fact, Keith had been told his progress was so dramatic that they were comfortable releasing him to the Brain Injury Day Treatment Program at Sacred Heart in Milwaukee to be under the care of its director, Dr. Jeffrey Cameron, which made my apprehension seem even more irrational. Keith was scheduled to be released after therapies on Wednesday, so Fred took the day off to attend therapies with him and bring him home that evening. In many ways I was excited to be leaving behind all the trauma we encountered in Madison, but I was also apprehensive about relinquishing the security of having easy access to Keith's doctors. I also knew I would miss Jason as there was a comfort in being embraced by his six foot, solid, healthy body. However, I was sure Jason was thrilled to have Keith on the road to recovery, and all of us on the road to Racine, so he could get on with his own life.

Wednesday nights I teach a course at Carthage College in Kenosha and the chairman of the department had been filling in for me. I was pleased Fred said he would be able to come to Madison so I could return to class. Fred and I were also very fortunate in that our school districts were extremely understanding and supportive of our need to be with Keith. Wisconsin has a family leave policy where we could take paid leaves using our accumulated sick days. Both our districts were allowing us the time we needed, and we were trying to balance our family needs with our commitment to the children in our respective school districts of Cudahy and South Milwaukee. I had officially requested, and was granted, a family leave and planned to be home with Keith during the day until he was capable of independent living. Fred never just assumed I would take the leave as parenting had always been a partnership. The decision was based on the fact that I was able to have a substitute teacher so service would continue for my students, while finding a temporary replacement principal posed a greater problem. Fred was still very involved with Keith's recovery, and all of us gained strength from his quiet demeanor and delightful sense of humor.

Oct. 17th: Fred, Keith, and I attended the first of many team conferences. At school I am frequently at multidisciplinary team meetings. The purpose of the team is to convey information concerning a child who has been evaluated for an exceptional need. With Keith I learned how uncomfortable it is to be the parent in that setting. First off, we too were outnumbered by the experts. Yet I have always felt, and it was confirmed by the year of the zebra, parents know their child best. All the data we were presented with was objective, but I discovered it is hard to look at your child objectively. In school we often offer suggestions of programs and placements to help a child succeed. What I learned is it hurts to hear your child needs those types of services.

Oct. 18th: (Keith) Today was a good day, a great day. Before I was released the doctor told me I could look forward to a wonderful life. Some people with MS never

CHAPTER FOUR

Sacred Heart Rehabilitation Hospital - Milwaukee, Wisconsin

Oct. 19th: When we left Madison we partially changed our base of support. Keith, Fred, and I would now rely on friends from the Racine area. Like Keith, most of his closest middle and high school friends had left Racine to attend college, so it was a "God sighting" that Matt and Andy who were recent graduates had accepted positions back in the area as they stayed close to Keith for the remainder of his life. Andy and Keith were not only good friends but also teammates since high school when they made it to the state doubles tennis tournament. Andy had also played with Keith when they won the 3-on-3 Hoop it Up Basketball Tournament in August. Matt and Keith shared a different passion and that was food, so it was appropriate our first night back in Racine Matt joined us for dinner at Keith's favorite Chinese restaurant following my class at Carthage.

At Keith's exit conference, conducted by one of Meriter's social workers, we were told he had difficulty with divided attention which meant he could not successfully process multiple tasks. They expected the problem to dissipate with time, but initially recommended we not leave him alone. Fred referred to it as shadowing him. I hadn't "watched" Keith for years, and it felt all wrong. The first time I understood what the doctors were telling us was when I tried to carry on a conversation with him while he was sorting through some of his mail. Mail was an upper for Keith. It made him feel good knowing so many people were thinking about him, and he always took time to read each and every message. In fact, he kept all his cards and letters in a large basket by his bed which he would frequently refer to at night. When I tried to talk to him while he was reading he became overwhelmed as he could not do two tasks at once. That freaked me because Keith was a multi-task orientated person, and I was used to him doing multiple things simultaneously like talking on the phone, snacking, listening to music, and folding his clothes. In the hospital setting he was somewhat sheltered, and only when he returned to his natural environment did I become acutely aware of the severity of his problems.

I learned that thinking takes energy, and that he would tire quickly from both mental and physical activities. Therefore, he was willing to have us do things for him and it was difficult to determine what was support and what was fostering learned helplessness. Keith was never good in the kitchen, so it was easy to laugh when he cooked his first pizza on preheat. Mistakes balancing his checkbook were not funny. Fred had tears in his eyes when he had to reteach Keith how to regroup doing subtraction problems such as 43-28. Keith was no longer comfortable with his mental math skills and was using a calculator. It also frustrated him that he couldn't write small enough to enter all the information on the lines in his checkbook. However, the biggest problem came when Keith asked me to enter his checks for him and my method just about drove him crazy. I do not believe in entering all the information the checkbook provides space for. Two out of four is enough for me to identify any check, so I might enter the date and who the check was to, or perhaps the number and the amount. My husband gave up years ago trying to change me and leaves balancing the checkbook to me, so after consultation with his father Keith also turned over his checkbook to me. Fred said that had nothing to do with fostering dependence, but rather trying to preserve Keith's mental health.

Oct. 20th: During the 26 years we had lived in the Milwaukee area I had driven by Scared Heart Rehabilitation Hospital on numerous occasions. With each passing my reaction was consistently a deep sense of sadness for the people needing the care found in such a facility. The thought of losing mobility is frightening to me and is the reason why I always wear a seat belt and bike helmet. It almost seemed surreal when I drove into their parking lot to admit my son, athlete, scholar, businessman, and from a mother's biased perspective just about perfect person, to their Brain Injury Department. This setting was different from the Madison hospitals as the entire complex was originally devoted to rehabilitation. At the time of our arrival they were in the process of moving the program to a new location so were in a period of transition, as were we.

Oct. 20th: (Keith) I went to Sacred Heart for the first time and met my recovery team. The therapists were really encouraging and referred to me as having a spontaneous recovery. I assured them I would be their most motivated patient and to expect to see a full recovery. The physical therapist recommended co-treating with the recreational therapist across the street in the gym. The thought of playing basketball again keeps me going. I fall asleep repeating PLAY HOOPS! My occupational therapist suggested I get on the Internet and research my condition. For starters, I need to buy a computer which I had planned to do. I'm scheduled for therapies four days a week and will meet the doctor in charge of my program Monday. My surgeon called today and said the report from Mayo's confirms the original diagnosis of Demyelinating Disease.

Oct. 22nd: I went out to breakfast with six of my best friends. In places near and far we are known as "The Baby Bunch." Seven of the eight of us met in the late sixties when we began our teaching careers at Park View Elementary School in Cudahy. The name "Baby Bunch" was bestowed upon us by the school secretary when Jan, Phyllis, Sue, Judy S., and myself were simultaneously experiencing our first pregnancies, and Karen was in the process of adopting her first child. Barb became an honorary member when we found out from her husband, who was our art teacher, they were also expecting their first baby. All seven of us initially chose to stay home with our children, so even though most of us are now teaching no one is currently at Park View. For over 25 years they have been my confidants, psychiatrists, parenting experts, marriage counselors, and spiritual advisors.

In the beginning we would get together for lunch once a month rotating homes and always taking our babies with us. We still meet regularly but at a restaurant, and now we also take an annual weekend trip in the fall. Originally we were a group of eight but in August 1994 Judy J., our youngest member, died of a malignant brain tumor. Within six months of her death Sue's husband suffered a fatal heart attack, and now one of our children had become seriously ill.

This morning the question of putting one's faith in God came up. I said I could not imagine losing my faith regardless of Keith's outcome. There is so much in this world that doesn't make sense to me that in order to function I need to put all my trust in God. I feel my view of life is short sighted, God knows the big picture, He is in control, and all things eventually do work together for good. I've always believed that, but now I knew my faith was being put to the test, and I was being asked to walk my talk. It did not take long for me to stumble for when I called home Fred told me Keith woke up with less strength and was able to do fewer exercises, and I immediately let worrisome thoughts take over in my mind.

Oct. 24th: (Keith) This was an interesting day. I met Dr. Cameron and he told me he felt MS was a highly unlikely diagnosis. He said one cannot make the diagnosis of Multiple Sclerosis in a patient with a history of only one clinical episode. I find the term MS unnerving so was relieved to hear a doctor say that diagnosis might not be definitive. I told Dr. Cameron that I was beginning to notice a slight increase in symptoms which I attribute to the reduction of Decadron and had contacted my surgeon in Madison who recommended I return to my previous level for at least another week. I notice I am walking with a slight limp.

Oct. 26th: (Keith) My boss drove up from Chicago today bearing good news. My latest performance review was such that I will be receiving a raise, and he assured me Quantum wants me back. We spent time hooking up my company computer so I could receive and send mail within the company. He seemed impressed with my progress, but I am fighting depression. I know I am losing more function each day. My speech is somewhat slower or at least word retrieval takes more time. I feel unsteady walking and can't walk longer than ten minutes due to a heaviness on my right side along with a tingling sensation in my extremities. Each day I'm doing less at therapy, but my therapists tell me to try and not become too discouraged as recovery is not always at a steady rate, and regressions are to be expected until the correct dosage of medication is determined.

Oct. 27th: The occupational therapist secured an article from the Medical College that seemed to accurately describe Keith's condition. The article reviewed thirty one cases of people who had large focal tumor-like demyelinating lesions on the brain similar in onset to Keith's. The article was positive because for the majority of the people in the study the lesions were a one time occurrence followed by a complete recovery. I was encouraged by the article, but very discouraged by the reality of Keith's current condition. It was hard to look at the fear in his eyes as each day he woke being able to do a little less. What was happening was not making any sense on a physical or spiritual level.

Oct. 28th: Again the weekend brought an abundance of Fred's family and friends to our home. Keith was having a great deal of trouble moving and you could see the concern on everyone's face. A fraternity brother and his wife spent the night, and before the three of them went out for dinner Keith asked me to join him while he was resting. For the first time since we left St. Mary's he confided in me how scared he was. He told me I couldn't imagine what it was like, and I knew he was right. I still can't fully comprehend the terror he must have felt as his physical and mental function was slowly being taken away from him day by day and sometimes even hour by hour. At the same time, I knew he could never understand how my heart was breaking watching him struggle to overcome whatever was sabotaging his brain. Our common bond was suffering made bearable by our love for each other.

Oct. 28th: (Keith) Today was a bad day. It was good to see my friends, family, and my fraternity brother, Jason, but I could not stop thinking about what was happening to me. The worst came when I went out for dinner. I found it hard to eat with my right hand, but I forced myself. At the end of the meal my arm began to shake, then I got hot all over, and had this impending feeling of doom. I asked to be driven home and was so afraid I was going to die before I could tell my family I loved them. When we arrived Mom and Dad were gone so I went to lie down. My parents returned shortly after and found me in my room emotionally upset. I wasn't scared to die, I just wanted to be able to say good-bye to them and tell them how much I love them. They assured me that they didn't think I was going to die, we all know of our deep love for each other, and whenever death occurs for any of us our love for each other will never be in question. Slowly I began to feel a little better. Dad said he would like to sleep with me which I knew he said so I wouldn't have to ask. I never thought at age 23 I would want to sleep with my father. When we went to bed we prayed and then spent time determining our territorial rights. He made me laugh, he's a good faith-filled man.

CHAPTER FIVE

St. Mary's Hospital - Milwaukee, Wisconsin

Oct. 29th: After a restless night Keith awoke feeling even weaker. Following breakfast his friends left, and I went to the phone. This was the second weekend in a row Keith needed to reach a doctor, and I was starting to realize how horrible weekends are for people with serious medical concerns. Neither his surgeon nor the neurologist who treated him in Madison were on call that Sunday. As a last resort I tried Dr. Cameron from Sacred Heart who had only seen Keith once. Dr. Cameron's expertise and responsibility was as his physical medicine and rehabilitation doctor, so I was not sure he could help us. He was on call, very concerned about the significant increase in symptoms, and asked us to meet him at the hospital. By the time we arrived, Keith was scheduled for an MRI. Keith was so weak that we had to transport him in a wheelchair to the proper department. Fred and I were again in the uncomfortable position of being in another St. Mary's waiting for test results. This hospital was newer but did not feel as comfortable as St. Mary's in Madison primarily because of where we were waiting for Dr. Cameron. Instead of being in the chapel we were sitting in a dismal empty hallway just down from the door to the morgue, looking at the stark reality that not every story has a happy ending. Dr. Cameron did not keep us waiting any longer than necessary coming to tell us before Keith was even back the MRI showed no new problem, but the original area was still enhanced which meant the demyelination was not under control. Later when Dr. Cameron met with Keith he was candid and forthright in sharing the limits of his knowledge regarding Demyelinating Disease. He told Keith he would be happy to be his Milwaukee medical quarterback but wanted to formulate a team of experts, which he successfully did.

What a difference from the first doctor we met in the emergency room at St. Mary's in Madison. Dr. Cameron did not give us any guarantees except the one we needed most which was the promise to access the best doctors and information available concerning Demyelinating Disease. For starters, he was able to contact Keith's neurologist in Madison who suggested Keith receive four days of IV Solu-Medrol, which is a mega amount of steroids. We were told the most effective way to administer the drug is in the hospital with 24 hour infusion. Due to admitting complications, Keith was given the option to up his oral steroids and return to the hospital Monday morning to begin the IV treatment. This would also allow Dr. Cameron time to secure other medical opinions.

Dr. Cameron became the most important doctor in Keith's life. Throughout the year of the zebra Keith personally interacted with 27 physicians concerning treatment options. Obtaining second and third opinions is wise, but 27 was overwhelming and often resulted in information that was confusing at its best and conflicting at its worse. So it was a "God sighting" Dr. Cameron always availed himself to Keith. He helped all of us gain an understanding of the implications regarding each and every recovery game plan recommended by the specialists. Often he would arrive with the latest research literally in his hands concerning the protocol Keith was considering. He constantly built Keith's medical knowledge base.

Fred and I tried to stay far removed from making decisions for Keith. We felt it was imperative Keith knew we would support any choices he made, but we did not feel comfortable making any recommendations concerning treatment. Consequently, Keith always drew his quarterback into the huddle of decision makers when a new treatment plan was proposed. Dr. Cameron filled the one role we did not want to take on by helping Keith understand his options so he could determine his own course of treatment throughout the year of the zebra. Keith valued their relationship both personally and professionally. He was the man whose judgment and integrity we came to trust above all others. However, as much as I learned to value Dr. Cameron's judgment, that Sunday I was apprehensive about bringing Keith back home as I was not sure he would be able to walk to the car the next morning. Keith made the decision to wait until Monday and spent the day at home with Joe, another friend from middle school, who had flown in from Washington DC.

Being surrounded by caring people was often the best medicine, fear was the only unwelcome guest in our home. Many times people would say, "Let us know if we can do anything." However, often we didn't even know what we needed, and the people we relied on were the ones who called with specific ideas. What we discovered is in times of crisis if you really want to help someone figure out the need and then fill it. Offers to visit, make a meal, take care of the lawn or dog were quickly accepted. Once a package arrived containing four dozen plants I had ordered during the summer for fall planting, and our neighbors spent an entire Saturday afternoon planting them for us. A few people were somehow selected as information gatherers and they would stay in regular contact. Their job was to dispense the news freeing us from having to tell the same story over and over. We also looked forward to the mailman delivering daily messages of support and encouragement. We appreciated both the serious and humorous cards. Keith's illness was having an impact on a much larger circle than our immediate family, and many people wanted to help which helped us. When we could not think of anything specific for them to do we would request that they just keep praying. There was no doubt we were being fueled by spiritual energy.

Oct. 30th: (Keith) This day reminded me of a scene from the movies where the frantic husband has to get his pregnant wife to the hospital. Mom was a nervous wreck. I was having significant problems, but was able to make it to the car with her help. Her anxiousness far exceeded the reality of my condition. Even Dr. Cameron had to ask her to relax when the drugs were not started immediately. Dr. Cameron requested the room with the best view which looks out over the park and Lake Michigan. From my vantage point I could watch people of all ages walking, rollerblading, and running on this perfect fall day. Life suddenly seems very unfair, and I wonder if I will ever be able to enjoy the great outdoors again. Less than two months ago I was backpacking in the Rocky Mountains, now I can barely walk. Another doctor, whom Dr. Cameron asked to evaluate my case, came over this afternoon. In his opinion I simply need more steroids to halt the demyelination. The steroids initially worked and in a higher dose they will be even more effective. He indicated there was a good chance I could use my airline ticket for Brazil over Christmas and return to work in January. His only additional recommendation was to extend the four day course of IV steroids to six. I can still go home Thursday with the last two days given in daily doses by a visiting nurse. I really want to believe this doctor, who specializes in MS, but am starting to get a sense why medicine is referred to as a practice. Mom felt better by the end of the day, and when Dad came she left saying she needed a month long bubble bath. We are settling in for a night of Monday Night Football. Dad is staying the night.

Oct. 31st: Trick or Treat? Initially receiving a 100% guarantee that nothing was physically wrong with Keith was a mean trick, but the quality of his medical care was a treat. Known for his wonderful ability to attract people with his infectious smile, contagious laugh, perpetual optimism, and quick wit Keith never lacked for medical attention. Keith was a shower person. He spent more time in the shower than any person I have ever known. At the Nabor House he would take a stool in the shower and just sit there until all the hot water was used up. Everyone who knew Keith knew he loved his showers. Therefore, he wanted regular showers at St. Mary's preferring more than one a day, which his physical and occupational therapists said he was too unsteady to do independently. So day after day he'd humorously convince staff to give up their breaks and stand outside the shower as he'd entertain them. One afternoon he even kept the MS specialist waiting until he got done with his shower.

Nov. 2nd: (Keith) Release day from my fourth hospital. This experience was brief but draining. Days were busy with therapies, treatments, visitors and working with Mom on my graduate school application, but nights were long and would have been difficult if I had been alone. Dad stayed every night which I really appreciated because the sheer volume of steroids make it difficult for me to sleep. When I do fall asleep, I experience dreams that come close to being nightmares. Steroids are nasty, and I look forward to the day they will no longer be in my system. Jason drove in from Madison to spring me from this place. As is customary for us, we had an adventure on the way home. This time it was a front tire blow out going full speed on the freeway. Thanks to his driving skills and my AAA card we were on our way in a short time, and I even felt up to going out for lunch. I'm moving much better, but certainly not as well as the last time I came home from the hospital. I agreed to bring home a stool to sit on while I shower which I hope will be a temporary situation, but said no to the cane. Sometimes I wonder if God's plan for me is to be a martyr. I can never deny the revelation I felt during surgery, and if I don't recover, on my deathbed I will still say God assured me I would be fine.

Nov. 3rd: A visiting nurse came twice a day to give Keith his intravenous treatments. I was uncomfortable having medical equipment and personnel in our home. I felt like they were invading my turf and there was no longer any place for me to go to get away. I have always had the motto I don't "do" illness. When Jason was small he had severe asthma. Fred and I quickly learned it was far better if he did the middle of the night emergency runs with Jason, while I remained at home with Keith and alerted the hospital of their impending arrival.

Fred is Mr. Calm and the boys benefited from that all their lives. We had a rule in our home that they could choose to ask either parent any question, but whatever answer that parent gave stuck. The only way they could get in trouble was if we discovered they asked both of us hoping for a different answer. It was not uncommon for them to tell us they had a question to ask and were taking their time to decide which one would most likely give the desired response. Only occasionally did we hear, "I asked the wrong one." Of course sometimes we would delay an answer saying we needed to take it under advisement with each other, but it did not take them long to figure out if they wanted to do something that involved some perceived risk, Mr. Calm was the man to ask.

Nov. 4th: My brother had flown in for the weekend to be with Keith, and he strongly recommended Fred and I take some time for ourselves. We had been one of the largest fund-raisers in the American Cancer Bike Ride and consequently had won a dinner certificate from the Abby, a resort on Lake Geneva. We chose to use it on that picturesque autumn day. For the first 50 minutes of the scenic drive out there we were oblivious to the scenery and totally focused on Keith when suddenly we looked at each other and asked ourselves what did we talk about before September 30th? We then made a concerted effort to try and take in the beauty of the colors and intentionally not mention the word Keith, but had to resort to reminding each other of our decision numerous times. We did discuss our plans to visit Nuria and Joe in Spain come summer. Now the last thing I wanted to do was go out of my comfort zone once Keith got better. For weeks I had been living in an environment that was foreign and uncomfortable. Consequently I had no desire to head off to a foreign land once this was over. All I wanted from summer was time to recover at home on my deck. Fred is the ever ready traveler, but agreed postponing the trip was a good idea. We did encounter another diversion that night when Fred was stopped for speeding. Our first date in months, and we landed in the snare of the local speed trap.

CHAPTER SIX

Sacred Heart - Milwaukee, Wisconsin

Nov. 6th: Our parents had offered to stay with us during the week and drive Keith to his therapies. Only months ago Fred and I were adjusting to being empty nesters and now we were contemplating having multiple generations under our roof. Without any additional variables that would have meant a significant lifestyle change. However, in this case, the variable drove our decision, and we correctly anticipated the benefits would far exceed the challenges. Stress was beginning to show on me in the form of significant weight loss. Consequently Fred felt it was important I get out of the medical environment and back into the classroom. I derive immense pleasure from teaching, so it was wonderful to be able to finally establish some normalcy in one significant area of my life. Children energize me, and it was therapeutic to be surrounded by hundreds of them freely moving their little bodies unencumbered by disease. When I walked back through the doors of General Mitchell Elementary School I could never imagine asking a child to sit still again, which lasted until after recess. Schools are a marvelous environment in which to view the goodness of life. To see the world through a child's eyes is to always experience the miracle of creation. I am fortunate to have selected a career where getting up for work is far more pleasure than pain, and something I look forward to each day. We had always stressed to the guys enjoying your job is far more important than the size of the paycheck, and to select a career with that in mind.

Nov. 7th: (Keith) I returned to Sacred Heart today ready to mount another comeback. Cognitively I am doing well which is amazing since I'm on a daily dose of 100mg of Prednisone. Tonight Mom and I worked on my essay for business school. My goal is to have it completed by Nov.15th. Mom is my recorder since I cannot write with my right hand. The word recorder reminds me of the words Dad recorded in my Bible Feb. 8, 1992. During college my parents paid for my room, board, and what was left of tuition after scholarships; books and spending money were my responsibility. Spring semester of the '92' school term I took "Archeology and the <u>Bible</u>*." Dad offered to purchase that particular textbook which was the* <u>Oxford</u> <u>Bible</u> *if he could inscribe it. He wrote, "Keith may your faith and family give you the support and strength to deal with whatever life may bring you. Love, Mom and Dad" I have those words memorized.*

Nov. 10th: (Keith) Saw Dr. Cameron today and he said he could not have hoped for more improvement. My right side is weak, but movement is returning rapidly. Mom, Dad and I went out for supper to celebrate, later Mom built a fire and began playing Christmas music. When I asked for clarification she replied, "Christmas could never be better than today, and from now on every good day will be Christmas." I must have caught the spirit as before coming to my room I made myself a cup of hot chocolate and brought along a Christmas tape.

Nov. 11th: We went to Madison so Keith could get the paperwork from his apartment that he needed to submit with his graduate school application. I had called Jason and asked if we could stop at his place for 30 minutes to use his computer. He suggested lunch first, but put us on notice he was still playing catch-up and did not have much free time. The first ice storm of the season had blanketed the city, and when I saw Jason helping Keith negotiate the ice it was evident how handicapped Keith had become, which seemed almost surreal since just last snow season Keith was skiing the black diamond advanced mountain trails. Our intended short and sweet visit turned into a long and laborious encounter of the most unpleasant kind. Keith was tired and discouraged that he needed help editing. Jason was on stress overload with his own school issues, and I was frustrated with the dynamics of their interaction along with being angry at the unfairness of the whole situation. After several arduous hours the application was ready for final copy. Fred and I left to visit Penny and Vern when the guys reconciled their differences and decided to go to Keith's apartment to watch a movie.

Nov. 11th: (Keith) I am getting so tired of needing help. Going from independence to dependence is incredibly frustrating. Today I responded with a variety of emotions. Jason is more emotional and has a shorter fuse than I do, and in the past I have been known to push his buttons much to my parents chagrin. Being thankful for his help, I have retrained myself to show restraint on those rare occasions when he irritates me. Today he was really ornery, and it took every ounce of my resolve not to verbally let him have it. In the past, physical exercise was always the way I worked off my stress, a couple hundred push-ups followed by the same number of sit-ups, and a few hours engaging in a physical sport that corresponded with the season kept me in good humor and head space. Now I have more stress than I have ever experienced in my entire life and no effective way to deal with it. It made me mad I needed his help, and he obviously resented having to give it, so it took forever for us to communicate effectively and get done. I felt bad asking for his help, and in the end he felt bad I needed it, so we decided to try and just forget about the afternoon and go hang out at my place for the night. When Jay and I arrived at my apartment I could not remember how to work my VCR which made me extremely angry. I yelled, swore, screamed, and kicked. Jason knew enough to stay out of my way, and I appreciated the opportunity to release weeks of pent up anger at an inanimate object rather than at the people who are helping me out the most. I also was grateful he told Mom and Dad everything had gone fine.

Nov. 12th: We met my mother at church. Her pastor had been a great support to us while Keith was in the Madison hospitals, so it was good to come to this house of worship as a family. The sidewalk leading to the sanctuary goes through the cemetery where my father's physical body is buried. Dad and Keith were very close, and I sure hoped Dad was doing all he could to help from his vantage point.

Afterwards we went out for breakfast and encountered a classic Murphy's Law experience. Not wanting to leave Keith's paperwork in the car for fear something unexpected might happen to it, I took it with me into the restaurant. Within minutes of being seated in the crowded restaurant the waitress spilled an entire glass of water narrowly missing Keith's application sitting on my lap. At that point I was saturated with people and problems, so following the meal suggested Fred, Keith, and my mom return to our home in Racine, saying I would take the application for final copy. What I didn't share was I really needed some down time. Jason wanted to go with me, which was amazing since I had already unexpectedly taken up most of his weekend. However, what he really needed was the opportunity to talk with me. That afternoon we both had hidden agendas. He poured sodas as he began to pour out his feelings. Both of us felt like Keith's illness was literally taking over our lives, and admitted at times we found that overwhelming. It was the first time I shared with Jason my fear that I did not know if I was up to this challenge. What I did not tell Jason that Sunday afternoon was I was really getting tired of putting on a happy face, and I could not fathom how Keith was able to keep that perpetual, never to be forgotten, smile on his face. Letting go and trusting God was feeling like no one was in control, and my spirituality was beginning a downward slide.

I apologized to Jason for the time I stole from him that weekend and reminded him how much we loved him. I stressed he was just as important to us as Keith, and he needed to make sure we were meeting his needs. He told me not to worry that he wasn't feeling like the left-back or never was. By the time we got to the copy store we were both in amazingly good humor. Consequently, we handled it well when the clerk told us we would have to do our own typing. Two hours later, everything was done, and those priceless pieces of paper were sealed in the proper envelopes ready for Jason to hand deliver to the Dean of the Graduate School of Business.

Nov. 12th: (Keith) Today I feel weaker, but want to think it is from overdoing this weekend. To others it might seem like I didn't do much, yet everything was an extreme effort, and I had to force myself to keep going. On the way home I asked Dad to stop at the store so I could purchase a thank you card for Mom and was able to write the message with my right hand. I am pleased my application is done, but feel a little sorry for myself and not quite as confident I have a future.

The following is Keith's essay for admission to the University of Wisconsin-Madison Graduate School for study in Business: Finance, Investment & Banking

The only constant in life is change. In August I met with Dr. Richard Miller to discuss my desire to pursue a joint business and law degree at the University of Wisconsin. Having already successfully taken the GMAT, I turned my attention to final preparations for the LSAT and writing my essays for admission into both programs. Sometime in September I wrote the following--I have experienced more in the last year and a half than most people experience in a lifetime. Little did I know how prophetic those words would become. On September 30, 1995, my world was turned upside down. Since that day each morning I wake up and tell myself that I am going to make a full recovery.

After four months of preparation and hard work I felt confident in my ability to score well on the LSAT, yet somehow I knew something was wrong going into the exam. During the test I became very confused. Unable to finish the exam, I canceled my score and requested to be taken to the emergency room. Forty-eight hours later I found myself in a hospital bed being told I had two brain masses and was going to die if nothing was done. The doctors informed me the MRI showed either tumors or an infection and only a biopsy would confirm the diagnosis. A craniotomy was performed the next day. Following surgery I lost all my speech and function on the right side of my body. Since that time my improvement has been miraculous. After sending the biopsy to the Mayo Clinic the correct diagnosis is an unusual form of Multiple Sclerosis. Doctors are confident I will make a 100 percent recovery within a few months, and statistics support their consensus that a similar episode will never happen again.

Since September 30, 1995, my perspective on life has changed, but not my desire to attend business school. With a global economy and rapidly developing technology in the work force, the job opportunities are changing so fast that I cannot pinpoint what I will be doing four years from now. I believe, however, that I can best prepare myself for the opportunities that will present themselves by furthering my education. While at Quantum, my inquisitive nature has been most intrigued by the financial aspects of my job. As a result, I am interested in pursuing a Masters of Business Administration Degree in Finance.

In May of 1994, upon graduation from the University of Illinois with a Bachelor of Science Degree in Biochemistry, I accepted a position with Quantum Chemical Company. I realized I was not ready for graduate school immediately after completing my undergraduate degree. I was not serious enough; not hungry enough. The maturity I have gained since that time is immeasurable. My job has required me to travel extensively between Cincinnati, Atlanta, Houston, New York, Philadelphia, and Orlando along with numerous cities in between. My responsibilities include innumerable business transactions with individuals from all positions in life as well as being responsible for millions of dollars of accounts. I have been provided with the benefits of being a young executive on the fast track, yet as I traveled from place to place I began to realize this was not what I wanted to do for a career. I feel the time is right to return to school. I look forward to the opportunity of earning my Masters of Business Administration Degree in Finance.

As American jurist Arthur Vanderbilt said, "Life has never been completely charted and as long as change is one of the great facts of life, it never will be." Unlike most of the changes my life has taken this fall, my return to school is a change I welcome.

Nov. 19th: I went to early church in Racine only to discover I was unable to get my emotions under control crying the entire service. My pain was for Keith and myself as once again he was playing the unwelcome game of How Low Can You Go. I have always believed that with enough effort, prayer power, and positive thinking any situation can be successfully handled. My children were raised to believe in God and themselves and trust they could accomplish whatever they were willing to strive for. Now my whole belief system was crumbling. Keith was trusting God completely and putting forth tremendous effort only to be met with disappointment upon disappointment. I was re-evaluating what the three of us experienced the day of surgery wondering if it was only wishful thinking or perhaps a figment of our imaginations, but I could not explain why three of us simultaneously had such profound and separate experiences. Nor could I understand how a supposedly good and gracious God could be playing such a cruel joke when even I, a mere mortal, do not make promises and then intentionally break them. Following the service Pastor Rusty invited me into his study where several others joined us for prayer. They prayed and I thought words, just useless words, falling on deaf ears, or worse, ears that hear but don't care. There was an emptiness in me I had never felt before, my Father had let me down.

We had only been attending Grace Baptist Church for a year before Keith got sick. Judy's death had led us there. She was the youngest member of the "Baby Bunch." I had stood up in her wedding, sat by her through 24 hours of labor, and knelt by her bed as I helped her plan her funeral. There was nothing we did not share, and we would often kid each other we would always be best friends because we knew too much about each other and would make dangerous enemies. Once she died a part of me died also, and I needed to go someplace where my soul could be rejuvenated and replenished. Perhaps by providence I was led to Grace Baptist Church, for it was there my spiritual needs and eventually our entire family's were met. I believe it was another "God sighting" for the same month Keith became sick Pastor Rusty came on staff as an associate pastor. Keith and Rusty became friends, and they learned from each other during the year of the zebra.

Nov. 19th: (Keith) I am going down faster than either of my previous rates of recovery. Tingling sensations have now moved to my left side. Jason calls every night, so being aware of how bad this week was offered to come home. Initially I said no, but this morning I asked Dad to please call and ask him to come. He arrived at noon in time to watch the Packer kick-off with me. I know he can't change anything, but his presence is such a stabilizer in my life. Dad and I are going to the doctor in the morning, and I'm glad Jay's staying to go with us. Mom is too upset to be put in a position of waiting for another set of MRI results. This will be my third one in seven weeks, and I am not sure if my insurance will authorize another $1200, so

I am prepared to write out the check myself as I need to know what is happening in my brain. My friend, Pastor Rusty, also came over this afternoon. Among other things we talked about Mom. I am afraid if I die she will become so angry and disillusioned she will lose her faith. I still believe God is in control where Mom isn't so confident. As a parent, Rusty says he can understand her reaction and not to underestimate the depth of her commitment to the Lord. Tonight when Mom asked what we talked about, she was startled when I told her. She assured me she would try to never lose her faith because that was what her entire life was built upon. I made her promise to always honor those words. She asked if it was payback time for all the promises I had made her like to look both ways before crossing the street, always wear my seat belt, and have a designated driver. I told her this was far more important than a life and death matter, it was a life after death matter.

Nov. 20th: (Keith) Dr. Cameron agreed to see us right away this morning. He spent about 45 minutes examining me and could definitely see a loss of movement on the right side. All tests on the left side indicated full function, but because of the significant loss on the right side he authorized another MRI which the hospital could not schedule until this afternoon. Dr. Cameron was going to be out of the office, so we had to leave the hospital without knowing the results. By the time we got home I was a nervous wreck. Grandma and Grandpa Kelroy who are going to be my chauffeurs for the week arrived just as we did and were shocked to see how my physical condition has deteriorated in a week's time. The phone was ringing as we walked in, and it was Dr. Cameron with the good news that the right side of my brain was not involved and the tingling must be the result of some cross-over sensations. Mom came home while I was still on the phone so I was immediately able to put her mind at ease. While sharing in my relief she kidded that for Christmas I should ask for my own MRI machine. Jason returned to Madison after supper, and Dad went to bed early suffering from what he termed the effects of an exhausting and stressful day.

Nov. 22nd: I had taken the day off to take Keith to the doctor. He was again sleeping with Fred because if he had to get up during the night he needed physical support, and we knew he appreciated the emotional support of not being alone when his mind just wouldn't let him rest. I usually fell asleep listening to them laughing over their territorial rights which were even more difficult to establish because the dog thought he should also sleep with them. Frequently I would wake in the middle of the night to the sounds of Fred in the kitchen making both of them hot chocolate. That morning I awoke to the discouraging news Keith was so weak we both would be needed to get him to the doctor. Thus, our Thanksgiving holiday began a day early without much to celebrate. Jason and Mom arrived that night. I clearly remember my mom sitting by Keith's bed reading to him as he rested just as she had read to me countless nights so many years ago. I thought grandchildren are suppose to be reading to and taking care of their grandparents not the other way around. My world was all wrong, and I was powerless to do anything about it.

Nov. 22nd: (Keith) I hit rock bottom. I was in to see the doctor who Dr. Cameron had consulted with when I was in the hospital, and he told me there was nothing more he could do. I will just have to ride this thing out and see how much, if any, I improve. My long term prognosis looks good. Steroids were working at high doses, but I can't stay on those doses because of long term side effects. In fact, the doctor wants me to decrease my medication. Fortunately there is no nerve damage. The right side works, and now we're just waiting for the myelin to heal itself which it does in four out of five people. I'm confident it will. The doctor would not speculate on how much I will get back cognitively or physically. My hand is clasped shut, and I cannot open it. I went out in a wheelchair holding a prescription for my own wheelchair in my left hand.

Nov. 23rd: Thanksgiving. In past years my biggest concern was where to seat and sleep everyone, or if dinner wasn't at our home how to transport food to assure it arriving at the proper temperature. Definite as Keith was about not spending the holiday in the hospital, he was positive he wanted to go to his Godmother's home which is about 70 miles north of Racine. All of Fred's family traditionally gathers on this day which is a highlight of the year. We are fortunate to be part of a wonderfully close knit family, like the Norman Rockwell painting.

That year Fred's sister Diane and husband Dave hosted the dinner, and there were 24 of us, including my mother. Keith was the oldest of 13 grandchildren of which twelve were living. Diane and Dave lost their first child to SIDS. Fred's siblings tell us we set the standard and we set it high for raising good kids, but it must run in the genes because each and every one of our nieces and nephews is great. We have had the delightful privilege of getting to know each of them by offering mini-summer camps at our house where we would invite them all to come and stay for a few days. We have some great memories of our train trip from Racine to Milwaukee to go to the museum, our day at the zoo looking for the zebra, visiting the state fair, making a campfire and roasting marshmallows by the pond, swimming, introducing them to the movie "The Princess Bride," kite flying, and best of all just having the time to get to know each of them personally.

What was happening to Keith was affecting everyone present that day in a very deep and personal way, especially his cousins. Following dinner, Keith did not encourage them to change to go out for the family football game as he always had in the past, instead they all gathered around him and watched a game on TV. Kristin and Amanda are twins and one of them had a dream they shared with Keith. I think it was Kristin who told him she dreamt his problem was he was just too smart and his brains could no longer fit in his head.

Fred supported Keith when he walked in and out of the house, I prepared his feast of food, and Jason assisted him when he needed to use the bathroom. Everyone noticed, but no one commented. The day unfolded as any other holiday with overeating, football games, multiple conversations, laughter, walks, naps, and the infamous late afternoon dessert table. After we left we found out Diane closed the door behind us and sobbed.

When we arrived home Keith wanted to play a game but not being able to use his right hand posed a problem. The guys came up with Blackjack and soon we were learning when to hit and when to stand. In real life Fred and I hit blackjacks with the birth of our sons, and for the most part enjoyed a 23 year winning streak. We had experienced some set-backs and a few significant losses, but overall had been very lucky. Now we were being dealt some bad hands, but to not be thankful on that day for the many blessings in our lives would have been to deny our past. We are blessed with a family that anyone would be proud to call their own, and we have never taken it for granted. Before Sept. 29th we enjoyed each and every year of our lives together, and our focus has always been on the family. Thanksgiving helped me remember that important fact. Regardless of what the future held there were no regrets concerning our past.

Nov. 24th: Keith was feeling stronger, so the guys took off for Illinois to visit Phil and Carissa. Christmas is our family's favorite time of the year, and the Friday after Thanksgiving officially begins the Kelroy Christmas season. Unofficially it begins in July when I play an occasional Christmas tape. We decided to follow tradition, and Fred and I took my mother out for lunch and shopping enjoying the hustle, bustle, and merriment of the day. It was that day I discovered I now look at people differently. Instead of noticing their outward appearance I watch their eyes and wonder what problems and pains they are carrying or have waiting for them when they return home. Life looks different without my rose colored glasses.

Nov. 28th: (Keith) Surprisingly with a reduction in medication I am making steady improvement. I'm again confident in my walking. Today I ate a bowl of cereal using my right arm and hand. I can move my right foot and ankle. Grandma and I decorated the Christmas tree in the living room. The top was mine, the bottom was hers, and the middle was up for grabs. Mom said hanging ornaments would be good therapy, and she was right. Once again I'm looking forward to see what tomorrow brings.

Nov. 29th: Several people approached me over the past several days inquiring if our family had seen a TV special that aired Thanksgiving night concerning a university student who two years ago experienced a sudden onset of symptoms similar to Keith's. Initially she was completely paralyzed and the diagnosis was a rare form of Multiple Sclerosis. She had returned to the university, but had to forfeit her volleyball scholarship. Keith definitely wanted to contact her. It was the first person he heard of that actually appeared to have a condition similar to his. She was about his age, and I think it was important for him to be able to connect with someone that actually had experienced something that resembled what he was going through.

Nov. 29th: (Keith) I continue to show physical and cognitive improvement. My arm movement is good, and I was able to brush my teeth using my right hand. Walking is easier. I went to therapy today and was able to walk on my own two feet throughout the day, but I am exhausted tonight. My vision continues to be blurry. It has been that way for two months. It has been one week now since I decreased my Predisone dosage from 100 mg to 80 mg. Tomorrow I go down to 60 mg. Hopefully, I've bottomed-out. Generally with a reduction in medication I start to feel signs of weakness, so tomorrow and the next few days should tell the story. Time will tell. I called a person my age who also has a rare form of MS, only her demyelination was in the spine where mine is in the brain. The main advice she gave me was to prove the doctors wrong. She said every time she could do something new the doctors would say that is great but don't expect anymore recovery. They never expected her to walk again, or even to be able to feed herself. There are two significant difference in our cases. First she never experienced any loss of cognitive ability, and once she was in the recovery mode she never had any setbacks, plateaus but nothing like I have experienced where I appear to go back to square one.

Nov. 30th: Our family room Christmas tree represents our heritage. The tree has over a thousand multi-colored lights that illuminate special ornaments that if they could talk would tell our family story. Because they can't each year we build fires in the fireplace, fill our mugs with hot chocolate, and become the voices of the ornaments as we relive and recall special events and people in our lives. The very top of the tree is reserved for ornaments we have received from important people in our lives who are now singing the refrain of "Angels We Have Heard On High" with the heavenly chorus. An ornament made by Fred's mom began the tradition with her death from cancer in 1978. She made the ornament during one of her long stays in the hospital. Having just turned six when she died Keith remembered Grandma for her hugs and cookie jar, a wonderful legacy to leave a grandchild. Then Jamie, a special student of mine, died of leukemia, and her homemade ornament was moved to the top. It was followed by one my dad had given us before his death from lung cancer in 1991, and finally last Christmas Judy's homemade ornament reached the top following a courageous battle with brain cancer. Fittingly it is a heart shaped ornament that says "Special Friend." Judy continues to bless my life. So many of the medical terms and procedures used with Keith I had become familiar with during her illness. As I viewed the tree, I was grateful for all of their lives and very happy Keith's ornaments were hanging near the bottom.

Nov. 30th: (Keith) Overall it was a good day. In general things are much easier to do using my right hand. Grandma and I decorated the tree in the family room. This is the fun tree where every ornament has a story. It's tradition Jason and I always move the ones around with our names on. It started when we played a game called The Christmas Game. The winner always got to put their ornament near the top while the losers had to place their ornaments near the bottom until the next game. So, we just carried the idea a step further and always try to put each other's ornaments on the lower branches. Grandma was unhappy I moved all of Jason's to the bottom of the tree, and after supper I found one of mine down there. Later Grandma laughed when she checked and found hers there instead of mine. I tied my shoes and shuffled cards. My endurance was up but it's the third day with a headache. However, we have begun playing Scrabble on a regular basis and even with a headache I am going to bed the champ.

Dec. 1st: Keith decided that he would not be able to return to his apartment in the near future and wanted to save the rent money. Fred was unable emotionally to handle the reality of Keith deciding to give up his apartment, so he stayed in Racine with him while I went to Madison to prepare for the movers. Keith's apartment was located on the far west side of Madison in a complex of about eight beautiful wood framed three story buildings. His apartment was on the top floor and was separated from the street by meticulously landscaped grounds. Last Mother's Day I spent with him checking out this apartment with my mom, Fred, and Jason. I remember the happiness we all felt for him as we unlocked the door and walked into what was to be his home for only a few months.

Now as I unlocked the door to his apartment, I realized what Fred meant. Prior to September 30th that key opened the door to a world of independence, built upon past achievements, current opportunities, and seemingly limitless potential. He selected this particular complex for all the amenities it offered. He did not mean the fireplace, cathedral ceiling, dishwasher or washer and dryer. No, he picked this address for its swimming pool, weight room, tennis, basketball, and volleyball courts. In fact, when he called Penny and Vern to tell them about his new place, the sports facilities were the only things he mentioned. They said that after his call they had absolutely no idea what his actual apartment looked like. Walking through each room remembering all the past joys and future hopes shared within those walls I became overwhelmed. From deep inside me, in a place I did not even know existed, a wail rose forth that I was incapable of stopping.

Dec. 1st: (Keith) Woke up with a serious headache and poor vision, my headache seems to increase as my vision decreases. Had another poor night of sleep. Cognitively I can remember what I read which is a far cry from when I took the LSAT on Sept. 30th.

Dec. 2nd: (Keith) Woke up feeling stronger, had the stamina to go Christmas shopping. My parents aren't so sure getting my brother a radar detector is such a good idea, but Mom can't say anything because that is what she is giving Dad. Poor Dad, no one likes to ride with him because he always drives the speed limit on the freeway, whereas we all prefer to travel whatever speed the fast lane is going. The problem with Dad is he likes 55 even on streets where the speed limit is reduced, so he is the one the officer wanted to talk with recently. This is the tenth day in a row that I've improved. My headache and vision were better. I read for two hours without experiencing blurry vision. I'm making a concerted effort to find out everything I can about MS. I read an in-depth study about people with MS which I previously read about a week ago and didn't comprehend whereas today I did. The problem is I can't read something and then explain it, but I'm coming along. My speech is really coming back, and I'm much more comfortable talking on the phone. I am going to fight this thing.

Dec. 4th: (Keith) Walked the whole neighborhood for the first time in three weeks and won at Scrabble. Both felt real good. Mom said since I'm such an intense player I might as well think about entering the World Championship of Scrabble. Actually, I'm using the game as an opportunity to reactivate my vocabulary, but being competitive by nature I do enjoy winning. I talked to Jason, and he is now busy studying for exams. I told him I was thinking about studying for the LSAT again. He said one of his professor's told him to tell me next time it won't be as big a headache.

Dec. 5th: (Keith) Once again I'm considerably better. I saw Dr. Cameron, and he used the word miraculous. My physical therapist said this is the best she has seen me since I have been at Sacred Heart. Played Ping-Pong today with my recreational therapist, he was just dinking the ball, but I was still hitting it back with my right hand. I came home from a full day of therapy, took a walk and then a shower standing up. No more stool. With all the prayers being offered on my behalf I believe this is it, and I am finally on the expressway to recovery with no more roadblocks or detours.

Dec.6th: (Keith) Took some concentration tests and that went really well. My wit is coming back, I'm becoming more spontaneous. Headache and vision were fine until after I read for two hours. I began writing a Christmas letter. Mom is big on thank you notes and I really am thankful for all the support I have received. Now that I am able to think and type, a general letter seems the best way to communicate my appreciation.

Dec. 7th: (Keith) Penny, Vern, and their daughter Julie came from Madison today. While Julie and I were watching the Packer game I discovered I can move my ankle in a circle which might not seem like a big deal, but it is when you can't do it. One lesson I've learned from this ordeal is there is a whole bunch I think we all take for granted until we can't do it anymore. I am now improving at a pace like when I first came out of surgery and should be doing great when we go to Kansas City for Christmas. There are great hills there for me to perfect my walk. I just got permission from my insurance company and Sacred Heart to stay out there for a few weeks. I have wonderful insurance, and my case manager, Timi McCauley, actually treats me as a person instead of an account number. She agreed after all that has happened the last few months I need a vacation. As much as we all care about each other I need out of here, and I think Mom and Dad will appreciate some time away from me.

Dec.8th: (Keith) What a day it was. Movers delivered the furniture from my apartment. I went up and down the stairs countless times and I could find the steps easily. My foot doesn't float in the air as much and I'm not having as much trouble placing it. Wrote out a check to the movers, and walked to the bank to transfer the funds. Mom teases me that unconditional love does not include paying my bills. I'm happy to have my own things here at the house. The downstairs is now my bachelor pad and workout room. I cannot imagine going through a medical crisis of this magnitude without good insurance and a strong support system. I am fortunate that I am receiving disability insurance and was able to return to my parents until I can work again. So far my medical bills have run over $50,000.

Dec. 11th: (Keith) I was able to ride a stationary bike at rehab for a couple of minutes before my right foot slid off as I have trouble feeling it. Talked to Dad about getting a bike. He says he thinks he can make something that would hold my foot in place, so we are going bike shopping. Went to the store to purchase some Christmas cards and have begun addressing envelopes. What a pain! Mom won't help because she says I have the time to do it and it is good therapy. My penmanship is horrible, but a friend of hers told me my poor penmanship is still better than Mom's. While at the store I showed Mom Sega Game Gear indicating it would be great therapy for

Christmas Letter

When things go wrong as they sometimes will,
When the road you're trudging seems all up hill,
When the funds are low and the debts are high

And you want to smile, but you have to sigh ,
When care is pressing you down a bit,
Rest if you must, but don't you quit.

Life is queer with its twists and turns,
As everyone of us sometimes learns,
And many a failure turns about when he might have won had he stuck it out:
Don't give up though the pace seems slow -
You may succeed with another blow.

Success is failure turned inside out -
The silver tint of the clouds of doubt,
And you never can tell how close you are,
It may be near when it seems so far;
So stick to the fight when you're hardest hit -
It's when things seem worst that you must not quit.

I read this poem every morning. And I assure you that I am not a quitter and
that I look forward to the day I can look back on this ordeal as nothing short
of a bad dream. The support and prayers I have received is unbelievable.
Usually one has to die to recieve support like I have, and then you don't get
to enjoy it. I have truly been blessed with wonderful friends and family.

I would like to share with you how things have gone the last couple of weeks.
We were in to see my doctor the Wednesday before Thanksgiving and that was
probably my lowest day as I was again basically unable to walk nor could I
move my right hand or arm. My Dr. informed me that there was nothing more he
could do and that he wanted to reduce my steroid dosage as I could not stay on
a dosage that high without risking long term side effects. He said that my
prognosis still looked good based on similar cases but he could not guarantee
me how much of my cognotive and physical abilities would return. The
realization that doctors don't know much about MS (multiple schlerosis) as
a whole and especially my presentation is probably the most frustrating aspect
of the whole disease.

Almost immediately after I received the news that my projected recovery was
pushed back from Jan 1st to 6 - 9 months I began to improve, which is ironic
because the doctor dcreased my steroid dosage. I want to stress the fact
that I know I'm going to get better and that I have a very positive attitude
about this whole thing. I know many of you are asking "Why Keith?". Why not?
No One made me the promise that life was fair. But I will get through this
though. And I will be stronger person for it.

I want to thank you again for all your prayers and support and ask that you
continue to pray for me. You will never know how much it has meant to me. No
doubt I could not make it through this trying time without it. Your support
has rejuvinated me and continues to give me the courage to fight.

P.S. NO MY MOM DID NOT TYPE THIS!!!!

Sincerely,

Keith

Dec. 17th: When Keith awoke he indicated that he felt weaker, and immediately I felt a lump in my throat and a pit in my stomach. I suggested a walk to calm my own emotions and figure out what to do, but Keith physically did not feel up to joining me. I went anyway and talked to God, actually I questioned him. For starters I challenged his wisdom creating Sundays as the day of rest when He didn't take into consideration how many medical crisis would arise on Sundays. A day of rest is a day empty of worries and what might look good on paper just did not translate into reality. I questioned the power of prayer as a healing force and the authenticity of His revelation. Then I got to the big one, "Do You even care?" I never denied His presence only His wisdom. So many questions, so few answers and to think I used to say so many malls, so little time. When I returned I relied on MY wisdom and told Keith if I was in the same situation I would return to a higher dosage of medication and contact my doctor on Monday.

Fred and I belong to an extremely caring and supportive small study group from our church, and that night the meeting was held at our home. Two doctors are members of our group which was another "God sighting" as they affirmed MY medical suggestion for Keith to up his medication, but they did kid me about not seeing my license on the wall. Actually the "God sighting" was knowing our prayers were always being lifted up through their continual prayer support even when I was too angry or exhausted to pray. A church some people humorously refer to as Grace Baptist, Catholic, Lutheran Church because a significant number of believers have come from those denominations, which makes it the right church for me.

Dec. 17th: (Keith) I have not had a headache for the last few days and my vision has been exceptional. I decreased my medication 2 days ago from 40 to 20mg of Prednisone. Now I'm noticing some right side weakness coming back. My walk is stiffer and it is harder to grip things. Going down stairs is harder. My hand wants to clench and remain clenched. It feels numb and tingling.

Dec. 18th: (Keith) I am back to 35mg. When I talked to the MS doctor, he told me that I can't cut that much and I feel pretty frustrated because that is the way he wrote out the prescription. Basically my vision is good and my headaches are gone, but my motor coordination is screwed up. This medicine is really touch and go. Today I had to use the shower stool again, and I can no longer eat with my right hand. Hopefully the 35mg will take care of my problems, and I believe it will. I continue to believe and trust that God is in control and I will be fine, and I am finding an increasing comfort level that I am in good hands in His hands.

Dec. 21st: (Keith) The 35mg has not kicked in. In looking back I think once the medication is dropped you cannot reverse the effects. That is bad news because it means I am going to drop until the medication is up to the actual body healing. I would not be comfortable going downstairs. My fingertips and toes are really tingly along with hot spots which are characteristics of other symptoms after a drop in medication.. I hate to guess how long this is going to drop downwards. Once again, we will just have to wait and see where the bottom falls out.

Dec. 22nd: Have medical concerns will travel. We certainly could have justified staying home for the holidays because of medical issues, but that's not our family's style. We've always tended to compensate for and overcome obstacles in our lives. My mom cannot fly because of ear problems and Keith needed more room for a ten hour ride than a car could provide, so we rented a van to transport the five of us to Kansas City. Each day Keith was waking up with less mobility, but he was still determined to travel. I called my brother at work, and we talked about making their house handicapped accessible and sleeping arrangements as Keith once again needed someone with him. We never discussed canceling the trip.

Dec. 23rd: Jason and my mom arrived. Amazingly, Jason had successfully completed his first semester of law school and felt confident his exams had gone well. Erroneously, I thought the professors would be sympathetic to his extenuating circumstances when it came to grades. Jason reminded me, in law school your entire course grade is the magic number you receive on the final exam. He said the professors were supportive, but for finals everyone is given a number to put on their exams instead of their names, consequently the professors are unaware as to which student's exam he/she is grading. Perhaps that is why there are so many jokes about lawyers without hearts, it's only the head that counts. Dinner consisted of Jason's favorite foods, and the games that followed were served with Jason's favorite snacks. That day Keith's needs were not my priority.

Dec. 24th: We had gone to evening church, followed by our traditional dinner and family gift exchange. It was evident presents do not make the season as ours was not the jolly holly house even as we sat among many unwrapped gifts that were on our individual wish lists, for what all of us had really wished and prayed for was not present. Even with filled stockings hung by the hearth the atmosphere resembled the Empty Stocking Club, and I felt like the Little Match Girl, using up my dwindling supply of faith trying to keep my heart from turning bitterly hard and cold. I had none of the good feelings of our healthy and happy Christmases past. It was essential, but not easy, that I look beyond the tinsel and gold to once again discover the real meaning of the season, and the meaning of my faith. I needed to go to the stable to stabilize my life.

Dec. 24th: (Keith) I am not doing too well physically. Vision is a little blurry, but no headaches. Cognitively I am still doing real well. I just can't figure out why this happened. Nine days ago I was walking two and a half miles, lifting weights with all my extremities, and now my right side is so weak and unstable. Tomorrow I am going to drop to 30mg of Prednisone and see what happens.

Dec. 25th: From the beginning Keith amazed me with his spirit, faith and determination. He kept assuring me that God said he was going to be fine. Keith had a gifted scientific mind, which made it impossible for his faith to be simplistic. Fred and I never wanted our children to go through the motions of a faith statement, when they were capable of understanding what they were saying, just to make us happy. Therefore we challenged them to search and discover their own faith while exposing them to church and our faith. To be confirmed was to be their own personal decision, not contingent on our expectations. Keith's scientific mind made his personal faith harder to come by. Often we had discussions about faith, and when he chose to be confirmed he told me it would have been easier if we had made him do it. I think it would have been easy for anyone going through what Keith was experiencing to become spiritually discouraged, especially someone his age. But as his physical strength diminished, we all witnessed a tremendous growth in his spiritual strength. While my faith had weakened to the warm glow of coals before going out, Keith was unconsciously, yet continually, blowing new spiritual life into me with his confidence and belief in God.

I have always prayed that my children would grow in faith, and God answered that prayer. Now I needed to recommit to my faith to get control of my fears. No one made me become a Christian. It was a choice I freely made, and it was time to trust that choice again and believe God was in control even though I felt like our lives were out of His control. I like the saying that God helps those who help themselves, and I have spent most of life telling God not to worry about me because I have things under control. It was humbling and healthy to admit this was not true for me anymore. Like the song, I had heard the bells that Christmas Day and a voice within me said, "God is not dead, nor does he sleep, do not despair this Holy Day new hope is born." Merry Christmas!!

Dec. 25th: (Keith) We spent the day with my Dad's family. I had anticipated being much better, so it was not my best Christmas. Tonight my brother helped me pack for our trip to Kansas City. Received a plaque from friends which reads: Lord Keep Me Strong! The blessings in the things we face come not from being in the race, but from the strength we have to run supplied in love by Your own Son. This is the hardest race of my life.

Dec. 26th: With the radar detector mounted on the window, we left for Kansas City. Jason rode shotgun, helping Fred understand all the flashing lights and warning sounds, my mom slept stretched out across the middle seats, and Keith and I sat in the back playing golf with his Sega Game Gear. All of us were content and mellowed out when the peace and quiet was interrupted by the continuous irritating sound of the radar detector. We simultaneously yelled, "Brake!" at which point Fred whizzed by the police car. Fortunately, Fred was traveling only slightly above the posted speed and the officer chose not to pursue our holiday green Christmas mobile. Fred was startled by all the commotion and only after passing the squad realized his foot must respond to what his ears hear and eyes see, which was a reminder for me that the real tangible feeling of God's presence the day of surgery would not be enough to see me through this life altering experience unless I responded with trust to what I felt. A trust Dr. James Dobson discusses in his book <u>When God Doesn't Make Sense </u>which Keith and I both read.

It is not difficult for some of us to believe that God is capable of performing mighty deeds. After all, he created the entire universe from nothingness. He has the power to do anything he chooses. Having faith in Him can be a fairly straightforward thing.

To demonstrate trust, however takes the relationship a step farther. It involves the element of risk. It requires us to depend on Him to keep his promises, even when proof is not provided. It is continuing to believe when the evidence points in the opposite direction...I'm convinced that faith in moments of crisis is insufficient, unless we are also willing to trust our very lives to His care. That is a learned response, and some people find it more difficult than others by reason of temperament.

Keith and I obviously had different spiritual temperaments. Keith trusted back in September, and I was tenaciously starting to trust now.

Dec. 28th: Empathy not sympathy was the mindset of all of us. Instead of physical activities like ice skating and family basketball games we enjoyed countless card, board, and video games. The Scrabble table was always full along with the cookies and candy trays. Keith somehow managed to keep his spirits up even though his physical function was going down, and none of us became Scrooge-like in our attitudes or actions.

Dec. 29th: (Keith) My right arm continues to lose function each day. My hand now is basically clasp shut unless I use my left hand to open it. Surprisingly my right leg has become stronger out here and I can manage the stairs quite successfully. I even walked a couple blocks this afternoon. Tonight I saw one of the guys I had gone back packing with in August for the first time since our trip. The look in his eyes was one of pity, and I tried to assure him that I am going to beat this thing. The more I think about this, I can't imagine living this way for the rest of my life. I am just to darn stubborn, and I have the rest of my life to get better.

Dec. 30th: Having had a good time during difficult times we left Keith in Kansas City and headed home. We were wrapping up the holidays. Gift giving had extended throughout the Christmas season as we exchange presents with our whole family and numerous friends. Repeating the ritual of giving those specially selected items, I began to accept in a new and healthy dimension the fact that Keith indeed was a gift from God. A one of a kind, irreplaceable, priceless gift that I treasured and enjoyed from the moment of conception, but he was not a possession. Whenever anyone talked about Keith they referred to his spirit, a spirit that was currently packaged in a very sick body that a mother's unconditional love couldn't fix. Yet God gave him to me with the same lifetime guarantee He gave all of us. I knew that when his physical body failed him, he would be given a new and improved version. Keith's spirit might not always be in the same package, but he would always BE! I never doubted that fact again.

Mayo Clinic - Rochester, Minnesota

Dec. 31st: I went through the mail and discovered Keith had an appointment scheduled at Mayo Clinic on January 17th. We could only assume that the MS doctor Keith was seeing in Milwaukee had requested an appointment but neglected to convey the information to us. I did recall the last time we were in to see him he indicated he was going to seek some additional opinions about the most effective way to treat Keith. With Keith continuing to lose function on the right side of his body that letter was a welcome piece of news, perhaps even another "God sighting" as Mayo's and miracles are almost synonymous. Fred said he was glad to see the year end because it had done enough damage to our family, and he was ready for a fresh start. We thought about burning the 1995 calendar, but were too tired to make a fire.

Dec. 31st: (Keith) Very hard day! We were supposed to visit friends tonight to ring in the New Year, but I just don't feel up to it. I guess there isn't any one thing that's worse, I just don't feel good. My Aunt and Uncle said they don't mind staying home, but I feel like all I am currently doing is ruining holidays. Hopefully, 1996 will bring better days. I just need to stay focused which is hard at age 23 as you never think something like this is going to happen to you.

Jan. 1st: We called all our children to wish them a happy and healthy New Year. Joe and Nuria, Morgana, and Jason were doing fine; Keith was worse. My heart literally hurt for him, it was a heartache as real as an ear or toothache. I believe what I was experiencing was the universal pain felt by mothers throughout the ages who have endured suffering with their children. Fred and I started to take down the holiday decorations which only added to the sadness building inside of me. New Year's Day was not a good day.

Jan. 3rd: Keith's problems were easier to deal with from a distance. Keith often told us we had no idea what he was going through. We agreed, and now I realized our support group had only a vague idea of what we were going through, experiencing something vicariously is not the same. People who said, "I can't imagine what you are going through," spoke the truth, and those who commented, "I know what you are going through" often didn't have a clue. It is difficult to describe what was happening in our lives. At the time I compared myself to being on the front line in a war zone, always on the alert for the next sneak attack. Time certainly was one enemy because as time was advancing movement was retreating from Keith.

Often the worse came after dark and each night we had to face the real possibility Keith would wake up with less movement. I do not know how Keith was ever able to rest knowing that fact. One day four fingers would open slowly, the next only three until within a week his right hand would be clenched shut. Those were the obvious changes, but the hardest and most painful for me was watching the sparkle in his eyes fade to a dull gray.

So with my brother Fred and sister-in-law on the front medical lines we were able to obtain some much needed rest and emotional recovery on the homefront as we always tried to be upbeat, positive, and optimistic around Keith. Daily reports indicated Keith's endurance was up but his right arm was becoming increasingly immobile. Keith was the reigning Scrabble champion, and the car automatically knew the way to the video store. He was never alone as Scott was on break from college, and they had become nocturnal sleeping during the day and staying up most of the night. Keith felt he would be able to attend the Chiefs play-off game on Sunday, and we decided to go to Illinois to visit Ginny and John. There is something safe and comfortable about old friends, especially friends who make you laugh even though they share your pain. Laughter is a wonderful cure for sadness.

Jan. 7th: (Keith) Today was a good day on the scale of good and bad days which is a whole new scale of good and bad days. Went to the Chiefs game and walked the total of half a mile or more. Only once did a guy have to ask me to get off his foot because I couldn't feel I was standing on it. Enjoyed the game, but it was mighty cold. Zero at kick-off which felt like I was back at Lambeau Field in Green Bay. It was hard to admit I needed help zipping my coat.

Jan. 11th: Fred called me at school during lunch to say my brother was flying home with Keith later that afternoon which was a week before his scheduled arrival. Keith had woken up with some right sided facial weakness and called his doctor who recommended he return home. My girlfriend Lori discovered me sitting at my desk, staring out the window, on that dark dreary day. My head was filled with wor-risome and fearful thoughts swirling around like the snow outside. I informed her of the latest medical update and verbalized how hard it was to watch Keith suffer from what I had unofficially named the Yo-Yo Syndrome. I shared the ups and downs were making me extremely apprehensive about the tomorrows ahead of us, but I didn't want Keith to sense my fears. She suggested I continue to interact honestly with Keith, but always hold out hope by reminding him God said he would be fine.

At the airport my brother and I walked arm-in-arm from the gate at which they arrived to the one through which he departed 20 minutes later. Before he left he told me not to give up hope. It was a two scoop hope day. The child in me wanted to run after him and be the little sister who grabbed his hand and he'd protect from trou-ble. Instead I waved goodbye with one hand and put my other arm around Keith's shoulder. Keith asked me if I thought he would be okay and the best I could respond was "I hope so because God told you so." Hope had to triumph over what we were experiencing.

Jan. 11th: (Keith) Woke up feeling like I had just returned from the dentist after receiving a shot of Novocaine on the right side of my mouth. When I looked in the mirror I realized the right side of my mouth was slightly drooping I tried to smile but after a couple of seconds my lip would sag. My uncle called just after I discovered my newest challenge, and he immediately came home from the office. By the time he arrived I'd reached my MS doctor who suggested I return to Milwaukee, and my uncle insisted on flying with me. I didn't need him, but he said he needed to do it for himself. I am really fortunate to have the family and extended family that I have, but it does get harder as it goes on. When we landed in Milwaukee I watched how all the other people unconsciously and confidently moved to exit the plane and I envied them. It is very tough to go on. I have to stay focused.

Jan. 13th: I came home from shopping just as Keith, Jason, and Fred were finishing up lunch. Inadvertently I must have been looking at Keith for he suddenly blurted out, "What are you staring at?" Then he began crying and said something to the effect, "I might as well get used to people looking at me as I look like a freak." Once we all regained our composure Keith shared how afraid he was, and we honestly told him we were also. The conversation that followed made it appropriate for us to suggest before he went to Mayo's he might want to fill out a document called the Power of Attorney For Health Care. The purpose of the document would be if Keith was ever in the position where he was alive, but could no longer make health care decisions for himself we would know what he wanted done in terms of treatment and care. In order for that power to be transferred to us two doctors' signatures would be needed to activate the document. It wasn't that we expected there would be a need for it, but for the last several months everything that was happening with him was unexpected. We knew we wanted to keep Keith in control, so therefore felt it was important that we be aware of what he wanted done in terms of health care in the event of a real crisis.

Jan. 13th: (Keith) Very hard day. I'm finding it tougher to go on. I'm living my life by twenty-four hour increments because that is all I can do. I need to get to Mayo's as the doctors here can't seem to help me. I realize every day is a day closer to death. Filled out my Power of Attorney For Health Care. I hope there will be no need to activate it, but I want quality not quantity of life. God told me I would be fine, I just need to stay focused.

POWER OF ATTORNEY FOR HEALTH CARE

FOR

NAME: *Keith Kelroy*

1.   NOTICE

You have the right to make decisions about your health care. No health care may be given to you over your objection, and necessary health care may not be stopped or withheld if you object.

Because your health care providers, in some cases, have not had the opportunity to establish a long-term relationship with you, they are often unfamiliar with your beliefs and values and the details of your family relationships. This poses a problem if you become physically or mentally unable to make decisions about your health care.

In order to avoid this problem, you may sign this legal document to specify the person whom you want to make health care decisions for you if you are unable to make those decisions personally. That person is known as your health care agent. You should take some time to discuss your thoughts and beliefs about medical treatment with the person or persons whom you have specified. You may state in this document any types of health care that you do or do not desire, and you may limit the authority of your health care agent as you wish. If your health care agent is unaware of your desires with respect to a particular health care decision, he or she is required to determine what would be in your best interests in making the decision.

This is an important legal document. It gives the person whom you specify broad powers to make health care decisions for you. It revokes any prior power of attorney for health care that you may have made. If you change your mind about whether a person should make health care decisions for you, or about which person that should be, you may revoke this document at any time by destroying the document or directing another person to destroy it in your presence, revoking it in a written statement which you sign and date or stating that is revoked in the presence of two witnesses. If you revoke, you should notify the person you had specified, your health care providers and any other person to whom you have given a copy. If the person you have specified is your spouse and your marriage is annulled or you are divorced after signing this document, the document is invalid.

DO NOT SIGN THIS DOCUMENT UNLESS YOU CLEARLY UNDERSTAND WHAT IT MEANS. IT IS SUGGESTED THAT YOU KEEP THE ORIGINAL OF THIS DOCUMENT ON FILE WITH YOUR PHYSICIAN.

2.   CREATION OF POWER OF ATTORNEY FOR HEALTH CARE

TO MY FAMILY, DOCTORS, AND ALL THOSE CONCERNED WITH MY CARE:

I, *Keith Kelroy* , *6500 Libra Lane* ,
    (Name)   (Address)

Racine WI 53406 being of sound mind, intend by this document
    (City, State, Zip Code)

to create a power of attorney for health care. My executing this power to create a power of attorney for health care is voluntary. I expect, despite the creation of this power of attorney for health care, to be fully informed about and allowed to participate in any health care decision for me, to the extent that I am able. For the purposes of this document, "health care decision" means an informed decision in the exercise of my right to accept, maintain, discontinue or refuse any care, treatment, service or procedure to maintain, diagnose or treat my physical or mental condition.

Keith Kelroy   *1-13-96*
    (Signature)   (Date)

3.   DESIGNATION OF HEALTH CARE AGENT

If I am no longer able to make health care decisions for myself, due to my incapacity, I hereby designate

Frederick or Karen Kelroy   *6500 Libra Lane* ,
    (Name)   (Address)

Racine   *WI*   *414 - 886 - 2960* ,
    (City, State, Zip Code)   (Telephone Number)

to be my health care agent for the purpose of making health care decisions on my behalf. If he or she is ever unable or unwilling to do so, I hereby designate

Jason Kelroy   *6500 Libra Lane* ,
    (Name)   (Address)

Racine   *WI*   *414 - 886 - 2900* ,
    (City, State, Zip Code)   (Telephone Number)

61

to be my alternate health care agent for the purpose of making health care decisions on my behalf. Neither the health care agent or the alternate health care agent whom I have designated is my health care provider, an employe of my health care provider or an employee of a health care facility in which I reside or am a patient or a spouse of any of those persons, or, if he or she is that health care provider or employee or spouse of that health care provider or employee, he or she is also my relative. For purposes of this document, "incapacity" exists if 2 physicians or a physician and a psychologist who have personally examined me sign a statement that specifically expresses their opinion that I have a condition that means that I am unable to receive and evaluate information effectively or to communicate decisions to such an extent that I lack the capacity to manage my health care decisions. A copy of that statement, if made, must be attached to this document.

Witness #2:

Print Name: _______________________________ Date: _1/15/96_______________

Address: ____

Signature: _______________________________

13.   STATEMENT OF HEALTH CARE AGENT

I understand that _Keith Kolrorg__________, has designated me to be his or her health care agent if he or
                               (Name of Principal)
she is ever found to have incapacity and unable to make health care decisions himself or herself.

_Keith Kelroy__________ has discussed his or her desires regarding health care decisions with me.
(Name of Principal)

Print Name: _Fred Kelroy + Karen Kelroy_ Date: _1-13-96_______
Address: _6500 Libra Lane Racine WI_____
Signature: _Fred Kelroy_ _Karen Kolroy_

14.   STATEMENT OF ALTERNATE HEALTH CARE AGENT

I understand that _Keith Kelroy__________, has designated me to be his or her health care agent if he or she is ever found to have incapacity and unable to make health care decisions himself or herself and if the person designated as health care agent is unable or unwilling to make those decisions.

_Keith Kelroy__________ has discussed his or her desires regarding health care decisions with me.

Print Name: _Jason Kelroy__________ Date: _1-13-96_______
Address: _6500 Libra Lane Racine WI_____
Signature: _Jason P. Kely_

Failure to execute a power of attorney for health care document under chapter 155 of the Wisconsin Statutes creates no presumption about the intent of any individual with regard to his or her health care decisions.

Suggested Language for the Special Provisions Section
of the Power of Attorney for Health Care Form

1. Life sustaining procedures, including non-orally ingested nutrition and hydration, may be withheld or withdrawn, if my agent agrees to it.

2. I do not wish to be kept alive on life sustaining procedures. My health care agent can determine the timing of the discontinuation of treatment.

3. My health care agent can make any decisions needed about life support procedures, including the decision to continue non-orally ingested nutrition and hydration and other treatment.

4. I do not wish to be kept alive on artificial life sustaining equipment, including non-orally ingested nutrition or hydration, if these procedures would only serve to prolong the dying process.

5. I do not want to be kept alive on artificial life sustaining equipment, including antibiotics and non-orally ingested nutrition or hydration, if these procedures would only serve to prolong the dying process or maintain me in a persistent vegetative state.

6. Non-orally ingested nutrition or hydration should only be withdrawn or withheld if my condition is stable and I am not expected to improve.

7. I allow non-orally ingested nutrition and hydration to be withdrawn so long as it does not affect my comfort.

8. Do not start or continue life sustaining procedures if my condition is stable and full independent functional capacity is not expected to return.

9. I wish no heroic measures.

10. If death is imminent, I want respiration discontinued and no CPR.

11. I wish no heroic measures, including 911 and no emergency medical services for life-threatening conditions.

12. I wish my health care agent to authorize all experimental drugs and treatment available which are supervised by a licensed health care professional.

13. I wish no (AZT, experimental drugs, experimental procedures, antibiotics, etc.) when my condition is stable and full independent functional capacity is not expected to return.

14. I wish no (AZT or other experimental drugs, experimental procedures) if these procedures would only serve to prolong the dying process or maintain me in a vegetative state.

15. I wish that only x, y, and z be permitted to visit me while I am incapacitated.

16. ˑ I authorize my health care agent to disclose my condition and prognosis only to my health care provic
and x, y and z.

17.   I would like my agent to keep ________________ informed of my health condition.

18.   I wish my health care agent to authorize all comfort measures, including narcotics, to the extent necess
to alleviate all of my pain, regardless of the possibility of addiction.

19.   'I authorize the use of all comfort measures, even those that will shorten my life expectancy and reduce
mental functioning.

20.   My agent may not donate my organs under any circumstances.

21.   I prefer not to participate in any organ donations.

22.   i would like to donate any body organs or medical tissue or blood that can be used.

23.   My agent can authorize organ donations and autopsy.

24.   Nursing home placement should be used only when home care alternatives have proved unworkable.

25.   I only want to go to a nursing home if no other alternatives are available.

26.   I would prefer not to be placed in a nursing home unless it is absolutely necessary and all community
resources have been exhausted.

27.   I only want to go to a nursing home if no other alternatives in the community are available.

28.   I prefer to not be placed in a nursing home or community based residential facility unless it is absolute!
necessary.

29.   I prefer to stay in my own home as long as possible.

30.   If consistent with my medical treatment, I would prefer to be treated at _St Mary's_ hospital.

31.   I revoke any prior executed Living Will executed on _____ (date if available). My health care agent ca
make the decision to withhold or withdraw life sustaining procedures.

32.   I authorize my health care agent to make all decisions not already covered in my Living Will so as to
cover those conditions where I am not terminally ill and/or my death is not imminent, as well as all
procedures not covered by my Living Will.

33.   Due to my religious beliefs, I do not wish to receive transfusions of blood or blood components.

34.   When I die, I wish the following arrangements to be made regarding my funeral

---

Adapted with permission from: Center for Public Representation, Madison, Wisconsin, Publication 9-90

4.   GENERAL STATEMENT OF AUTHORITY GRANTED

Unless I have specified otherwise in this document, if I ever have incapacity I instruct my health care provider to obtain the health care decision of my health care agent for all of my health care. I have discussed my desires thoroughly with my health care agent and believe that he or she understands my philosophy regarding the health care decisions I would make if I were so able. I desire that my wishes be carried out through the authority given to my health care agent under this document.

My health care agent is instructed that if I am unable, due to my incapacity, to make a health care decision he or she shall make a health care decision for me, except that in exercising the authority given to my health care agent under this document.

My health care agent is instructed that if I am unable, due to my incapacity, to make a health care decision, he or shall make a health care decision for me, except that in exercising the authority given to him or her by this document, my health care agent should try to discuss with me any specific proposed health care if I am able to communicate in any manner, including by blinking my eyes. If this communication cannot be made, my health care agent shall base his or her health care decision on any health care choices that I have expressed prior to the time of the decision. If I have not expressed a health care choice about the health care in question and communication cannot be made, my health care agent shall base his or her health care decision on what he or she believes to be in my best interest.

5.   LIMITATIONS ON MENTAL HEALTH TREATMENT

My health care agent may not admit or commit me on an inpatient basis to an institution for mental diseases, an intermediate care facility for the mental diseases, an intermediate care facility for the mentally retarded, a state treatment facility or a treatment facility. My health care agent may not consent to experimental mental health research or psychosurgery, electroconvulsive treatment or other drastic mental health treatment procedures for me.

6.   ADMISSION TO NURSING HOMES OR COMMUNITY-BASED RESIDENTIAL FACILITIES

My health care agent may admit me to a nursing home or community-based residential facility for short-term stays for recuperative care or respite care.

If I am diagnosed as mentally ill or developmentally disabled, my health care agent may not admit me to a nursing home or community-based residential facility for a purpose other than recuperative care or respite care.

If I am not diagnosed as mentally ill or developmentally disabled, and if I have checked "Yes" to the following, my health care agent may admit me for a purpose other than recuperative care or respite care to:

(1)   A nursing home   ____YES   ____NO

(2)   A community-based
residential facility   ____YES   ____NO

If I have not checked either "Yes" or "No" to admission to a nursing home or community-based residential facility for a purpose other than recuperative care or respite care, my health care agent may only admit me for short-term stays for recuperative care or respite care.

7.   PROVISION OF NONORALLY INGESTED NUTRITION AND HYDRATION

If I have checked "Yes" to the following, my health care agent may have nonorally ingested nutrition and hydration withheld or withdrawn from me, unless my physician has advised that, in his or her professional judgement, this will cause me pain or will reduce my comfort. If I have checked "No" to the following, my health care agent may not have nonorally ingested nutrition and hydration withheld or withdrawn from me.

Withhold or withdraw nonorally ingested nutrition and hydration   ✓ YES   ____NO

If I have not checked either "Yes" or "No" to withholding or withdrawing nonorally ingested nutrition and hydration, my health care agent may not have nonorally ingested nutrition and hydration withdrawn from me.

8.   HEALTH CARE DECISIONS FOR PREGNANT WOMEN

If I have checked "Yes" to the following, my health care agent may make health care decisions for me even if my agent knows I am pregnant. If I have checked "No" to the following, my health care agent may not make health care decisions for me if my health care agent knows I am pregnant.

Health care decision if I am pregnant   ____YES   ____NO

If I have checked either "Yes" or "No" to permitting my health care agent to make health care decisions for me if I am known to be pregnant, my health care agent may not make health care decisions for me if my health care agent knows I am pregnant.

9.   STATEMENT OF DESIRES, SPECIAL PROVISIONS OR LIMITATIONS

In exercising authority under this document, my health care agent shall act consistently with my following stated desires, if any, and is subject to any special provisions or limitations that I specify. The following are any specific desires, provisions or limitations that I wish to state (add more items if needed):

(1) _Please give special attention to numbers 2-5-8-19-22 + 23 on suggested language for this section - see_

(2) _attached sheets_
Basicly - No heroics - don't continue treatment if full independent

(3) _functional capacity is not expected to return and my organs can be donated - Drivers license is signed_

10.   INSPECTION AND DISCLOSURE OF INFORMATION RELATING TO MY PHYSICAL OR MENTAL HEALTH

Subject to any limitations in this document, my health care agent has the authority to do all of the following:

(1)   Request, view and receive any information, verbal or written, regarding my physical or mental health, including medical and hospital records.

(2)   Execute on my behalf any documents that may be required in order to obtain this information.

(3)   Consent to the disclosure of this information.

11.   SIGNING DOCUMENTS, WAIVERS AND RELEASES

Where necessary to implement the health care decisions that my health care agent is authorized by this document to make, my health care agent has the authority to execute on my behalf any of the following:

(1)   Documents titled or purporting to be a "Consent Permit Treatment," "Refusal to Permit Treatment" or "Leaving Hospital Against Medical Advice."

(2)   A waiver or release from liability required by a hospital or physician.

12.   STATEMENT OF WITNESSES

I know the principal personally and I believe him or her to be of sound mind and at least 18 years of age. I believe that his or her execution of this power of attorney for health care is voluntary. I am at least 18 years of age and am not related to the principal by blood, marriage or adoption. I am not a health care provider who is serving the principal at this time. To the best of my knowledge, I am not entitled to and do not have a claim on the principal's estate.

Witness #1:
Print Name:_______________________________   Date: 1-13-96

Address:____

Signature:_______________________________________

Jan 17th: (Keith) Dad and I are here at Mayo's. He said he felt like the mailman driving me here through ice, snow, sleet, and hail. Tonight there is such a blizzard in progress we cannot see across the street. Our room is in an old hotel directly across from the Mayo clinic which is good because it is hard for me to walk. I'm beginning to have trouble with word retrieval, and I think my speech is affected, but Dad says he can't hear it. It is taking me longer to say what I want to say and part of my tongue feels numb. My strength continues to come from my faith and family. I am a pretty strong person, and I will fight this to the end. At least that's the way I feel tonight.

Jan. 18th: (Keith). Saw several doctors today and had another MRI that showed enhancement which confirms the demyelination is active. What I have looks like MS, but is not responding like it traditionally would. The doctors told me my problem is so unusual that it could be classified as one in a million. They are recommending that I begin another round of IV Solu-Medrol and if that doesn't halt the process enter a government study involving plasmapheresis which is a blood filtration treatment. They suggested starting treatment tonight, but I wanted an opportunity to talk to my MS specialist in Milwaukee and Dr. Cameron which I just did. They thought I should agree to another round of steroids. I hate what steroids do to me, and I am worried about long term side effects. The doctors all feel I can't worry about long term side effects until I get the immediate problem under control which is halting the demyelination. Dad is leaving the decision up to me. He went to find us some food while I'm taping. There is so much snow they are removing it with dump trucks. It is hard for me to get around, and I hate the thought that a wheelchair is outside my door. I'm keeping my attitude up trying to stay focused on what I can do because what I can't do changes from day to day. I can still beat Dad at Scrabble.

Jan. 19th: It was a strange week. Jason was in Florida, Fred and Keith were in Rochester, and I was home alone. The news from Rochester was not encouraging. Keith was definitely experiencing aggressive demyelination that was not responding to traditional treatment. Pastor Rusty came and brought a doctor to listen and pray with me as I tried to understand God's will in all of this. I told Pastor Rusty I was so confused by everything that was happening I could not begin to discern God's will or purpose in any of it. He told me we were all in a survival mode and it was okay to leave the praying to others. Just getting up and facing each day took courage and was all that was expected at this point. While they were here, Fred called and said Keith would be receiving his first treatment unless I had any reason why he shouldn't. The doctor agreed it sounded like the best course of action, but also said Keith's condition was so serious we were now in the realm of needing a miracle. Thinking the outcome was in God's hands was both scary and comforting as there was no doubt it was out of my control. In some ways it was a relief knowing there was nothing more I could be doing to help Keith, yet I kept thinking God could be doing a lot more.

Jason returned from his trip with the news he had decided not to return to law school because he wanted to see this through with Keith. I responded with mixed emotions. I hated the thought of him putting his dreams on hold, but knew we would benefit from his priceless gift of presence. All of his life we have called Jason the family's greatest fan. He's the family cheerleader and was Keith's best friend. I asked him to wait to make the final decision until he saw Keith which would be the next day.

Jan. 20th: Fred and Keith left for Rochester Minnesota with maps and directions and were pleased they only made one wrong turn while Jason and I made the 300 mile trip with just the name of the hotel, the Colonial Inn, and drove directly to the entrance. The difference in our directionality ability became even more humorous when Fred said that if Keith would return for plasmapheresis he would receive treatment at a facility called the Hilton. Fred had rented another room for our family that night which was at the end of the floor they were staying on and its window faced the side street. We were all in that room when Fred suggested we might want to locate the Hilton and select where we would stay in regard to that location should Keith decide to enter the study. Fred and Keith had already been at Mayo's four days when he pulled out the map to determine the exact location of the Hilton. As he was mentioning the roads, Jason and I began to smile and Jason went to the window. Directly across the street in huge block letters was the word HILTON. Fred and Keith couldn't believe it, and Jason referred to them as "hopeless."

Later, we went with Keith to Methodist Hospital via the maze of underground tunnels watching Jason pop wheelies with Keith in the wheelchair. He was receiving his second of five IV treatments and was impressed that they numbed the area on his arm before inserting the needle which was the only hospital that extended that courtesy. While he received his treatment we all played Scrabble. During dinner, Jason and Keith discussed the idea of Jason deferring law school for one semester. Keith confirmed that he really enjoyed Jason's companionship. However, Keith did not want to feel responsible or guilty for asking Jason to stay with him. Keith really wanted Jason to do what was best for Jason. I understood the dilemma Jason was facing. What would be best for him was for Keith to be well and both of them living happily in Madison. He wanted something he could not have which was peace of mind and clarity of direction. He wanted to be with Keith, and he wanted to return to school. Like all of us, he was caught in the web of making unhappy and difficult choices.

Jan. 21st: Jason was still unsure of his decision. I told him that I did not think he would ever regret staying home for one semester, but I could not say the same would be true if he went to school. Jason is a worrier and he does worry about all of us. Therefore I felt even if he enrolled in school what was happening in our lives would constantly impact on his ability to study and concentrate. I knew if Keith continued to have problems Jason would want to try and be part of the solution. The future was so uncertain none of us could predict what even tomorrow would bring. If he did stay the three of us would be winners as we all enjoyed having him around. When Keith and Jason were together it was very hard to be serious because they really were a comedy team. But I did not think Jay should stay if it would make him feel like a loser by giving up something so important to him. He said he just needed to hear we really wanted him. Apparently by our showing hesitancy he was perceiving it as we thought it might be better if he wasn't around, which was far from the truth. Suddenly I was overwhelmed with the depth of his love for our family. At age 21 I could not have made the same decision. In fact I would have been relieved to have a legitimate reason not to stay. Even now there was still a part of me that wanted to run far far away. After lunch we went our separate ways. Jason and I turned east toward Wisconsin while Fred and Keith headed west to Methodist Hospital for another treatment.

On the way home we decided the easiest way to communicate the latest news to our family and friends would be through a letter. I took the wheel while Jason typed on the keys of his laptop computer. Deciding what to write gave us time to review and reflect on the information we had received concerning treatment options. We knew no definite solutions were available for Keith's problems and acknowledged that was not good news. The challenge we were facing was to find a way to communicate that fact to our family and friends in a positive manner. By the time we reached the printer at his apartment we had come to terms with the seriousness of Keith's condition. Jason needed to spend the night in Madison in order to officially withdraw from school the next day. I left him the car and my luggage so he could pack up some of his clothes, and took the bus to Milwaukee.

My friend Lori picked me up and couldn't stop laughing as I walked up to her car carrying my belongings in a garbage bag. She told me to get in and tell her how I had become the "Bag Lady." Laughing and crying at the same time I told her, "I'm down on my luck, going through some hard times, and can you lend me a buck?" On the way to Racine we stopped at Fred's superintendent's house to drop off a copy of our newsletter.

Our letters were being distributed throughout both school districts and among our large circle of friends. So many people were communicating with us that it was impossible to keep up on an individual basis. Yet we wanted people to know that their support was making a positive difference in our ability to cope. We never took it for granted that people were taking time out of their busy lives to make ours easier. Sometimes just knowing that people were watching to see how I was going to handle the latest crisis gave me the strength I needed to deal with it. God knows our family never asked to be cast in this real life drama, but once we were I wanted to play my role well. Many people did impact and change our lives on a daily basis by their selfless acts of kindness.

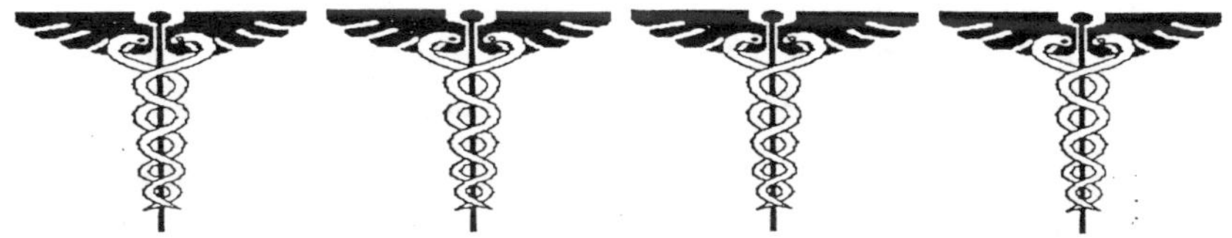

4:00 Sunday evening, in the car on the way home from Mayo Clinic:

Medical Update From The Kelroys

Appreciating the fact that so many of you have shown concern over Keith, I thought that the easiest way to update you would be through this correspondence. As I drive, and Jason takes dictation, Fred is with Keith as he receives his third intravenous treatment of a five day program. I wish I could give you answers about what is going on in Keith's brain, but even the very best doctors at Mayo cannot give them to us. We do know that Keith is having aggressive demyelination that up until this point as been unable to be stopped. Currently, he has no movement of his right arm, limited use of his right leg, cognitive involvement, and some paralysis of the right side of his lips and tongue. As dismal as that sounds, his personality and faith are still in place and he continues to give us great joy.

After consultation with the doctors, Keith decided to undergo aggressive treatment in hopes of halting and possibly even reversing the demyelination process. There are two specific medical protocols, one of which Keith is already undergoing, and a second which will be utilized based on Keith's response to the first one. Although the demyelination mimics MS and the treatment options are based on treatments for MS, the doctors feel that this is not MS but rather Keith has been exposed to some undetermined infectious agent. Therefore, without knowing the cause, it is difficult to come up with a treatment and even more difficult to predict the outcome. In one doctor's words, we need a miracle.

Jason has made the decision to postpone his return to law school this semester in order to support his brother and us in any way he can. As difficult as it was to realize that the situation is this serious, we know that Jason's decision is the best for everyone. With Jason's help, Fred and I will be able to be at school just as much as we possibly can. At this point, Fred is still at Mayo's with Keith and plans on being back at work on Thursday. If Keith needs to return to Mayo for another round of treatments, Jason and I are planning on being with him.

We are continually humbled by how many people ask how they can help. Prayers, mail, and moral support are what we need most. Keith values knowing that people care about him.

Not to leave you on a down note, the four of us did have some very good times this weekend. At dinner our waitress commented on what wonderful sons we had and what a special family we appeared to be. That was even after Keith had just beat us in Scrabble, which we played while he received his IV treatment, by using all seven letters creating the word "saviors." Our faith continues to bring us comfort and joy (and Keith points) in many countless ways. Earlier the doctors told Keith that (medically) he was one in a million, which did not surprise us as we have always felt that our family was one in a million.

Thank you for caring about us,

Karen

Jan. 22nd: I could not believe Fred and Keith were traveling on bad roads again. I was glad the car had a phone as I knew Keith would have been unable to walk any distance in case of trouble. When Fred called and said they had made it to my mom's I heard the exhaustion in his voice. He said Keith really wanted to come home, so after some coffee they planned on trying to make it the rest of the way. I asked if he was willing to stay if I could convince Keith, and he wearily replied, "Yes," which told me he had fought the roads and weather long enough as Fred prefers to sleep in his own bed whenever possible. When Keith got on the phone, I realized he wasn't so concerned about getting home that night as he was about the fact Fred would want to get up and come home bright and early, a phrase not in Keith's vocabulary. I told him Jason was in Madison so he could sleep in, and Jay would bring him home whatever time he wanted to come. I also reminded him I am a worrier by nature, and knowing they were safe on such a stormy night was better than being able to physically see them, which he knew I had been counting on. He reluctantly agreed.

Jan. 22nd: (Keith) After my last treatment, Dad and I met again with my doctors who said we had to wait and see if the steroids will work. I don't think they will as I haven't noticed any change. We left Rochester during another snow storm. Dad needed my help because there were so many white outs he had trouble seeing the road. Once I told him to move to the right, and we almost went in the ditch because I confused my right and left. We laughed, but knew Mom wouldn't have found it funny. Most likely we would have found her on the floor from total fear if she had been in the car. After that I tried to use words like middle and edge, but saying those quick enough was sometimes hard. Cognitively I'm slow and my vision is blurry, so I really had trouble seeing with the blowing snow and wasn't much help. It is bullshit what happened to me. Didn't have any trouble getting that word out. We did not arrive at Grandma's until after ten tonight. It took five and a half hours to drive 200 miles. I really want to get home to my dog Sam and bed, but when I talked to Mom she asked us to please stay over so she wouldn't stay up and worry. She is the Queen of Worry.

Jan. 23rd: Fred had gotten up early, which Keith had correctly anticipated, and headed for home. When I arrived home after school Keith and Jason were also there. Fred said that he was so emotionally wiped out that all he did was wander around the house being totally unproductive. I felt guilty because I had sent Fred alone to Rochester with Keith. I told him I just couldn't handle the initial evaluation that was going to be done at the Mayo Clinic. For me, waiting for news was always the hardest part. Once I knew the diagnosis and course of treatment I was able to "get a grip," as the guys would say. At the time Fred said he understood. He reminded me that he couldn't pack up Keith's apartment, but he could and would take Keith to

Mayo's. I know it was harder on him than he anticipated just as doing Keith's apartment was harder on me than I thought it would be. I told Fred I was preparing to return to Rochester with Keith and Jason if this treatment didn't work. Keith looked even more emotionally and physically drained than Fred. His sunken eyes were surrounded by dark circles, his lower lip continued to droop, and it appeared he had lost a significant amount of weight. I wanted to pick him up in my arms and rock him, rock him, rock him. Instead we played Scrabble, and I lost.

Jan. 23rd: (Keith) It was a pretty good day. Some enjoyment out of life today. Feels real good to be home with my family and Sammy. You can either get busy dying or living. I chose to get busy living. I just keep trusting the Lord.

Jan. 24th: Fred went off to work looking incredibly frumpy wearing a dull baggy sweater and plain pants. He is an extremely handsome suit and tie man, so the way he dressed for his first day back at work in over a week was totally out of character. I was very worried about him. When he came home that night he told me he felt like crying or throwing up the entire day. I suggested a walk, and holding tightly onto his hand that cold starlit night I tried to melt his despair. Fred is Mr. Fix-it. We all take our real, or imaginary problems to him, and he can always make things better. This time he had to realize, and believe, none of us expected him to fix this, not Keith, certainly not Jason or I, and not even God. I reminded him that our family had always been his first priority, and no father or husband could do more than what he had always done which was to be there for all of us. The next morning, and every morning thereafter, Fred went out the door looking very dapper. Thanks to Jason that was the first and last time only one of us stayed alone with Keith at Rochester for any extended time.

Jan. 27th: Jeff, another fraternity brother, arrived who was working on a project over in the Ukraine through the University of Illinois and was currently home for the holidays. Keith had leveled out, but was not noticing any dramatic improvement so we all were mentally preparing to return to Mayo's on Wednesday. Therefore, it was good to have someone else in the house for a few days to help divert our worrisome thoughts with positive activities. Keith appeared to become even more determined to get well, especially when they talked about their adventures from days gone by, such as when they were driving and the steering wheel of the car literally fell off as they rounded a corner.

Jan. 29th: (Keith) Was sorry to see my friend leave. Tonight I want to beat this thing, and I am going to beat this thing no matter how long it takes. That is how I feel tonight. And another thing, as long as I am alive I will keep fighting. I will not continue to doubt that I will get well. I want to dribble a basketball so bad again that I can taste it. I will not quit or believe I will not get better.

Jan. 30th: Fred's brother Tom and his wife Gloria came to spend the day with us. We joked with Keith that at least he could have come up with the type of unusual problem that needed to be addressed at the Mayo Clinic in warm and sunny Arizona. The cold reality was the warmth of family, friends, fireplaces, and familiar places were to be left behind at the close of this day.

Jan. 30th: (Keith) No dramatic improvement. Emotionally a good day. I am ready to go back to Mayo's. I want my life back, so I will do all I can to get well. I will continue to fight this thing, and I will get well.

CHAPTER EIGHT

Mayo's - Rochester, Minnesota

Jan. 31st: Jason, Keith, and I traveled back to Mayo's on a bitterly cold sunny day. The only difficulty we encountered was changing lanes on the expressway. Each crossing was like driving over a speed bump due to the build-up of ice in the center caused by temperatures so low salt was rendered ineffective. We arrived to discover expected actual temperatures were about 40 degrees below zero, but with no cooking facilities in our room we were forced to venture out to a restaurant, and not surprisingly we found it basically deserted so enjoyed a quiet dinner with great service. Afterwards, I lost in Scrabble while hovering under blankets drinking steaming hot chocolate. Our room at the Colonial Inn was due for renovation, so the price was right. However that meant dreary furnishings, window treatments that were ragged and torn, and inadequate lights that were little more than bare bulbs. Our living conditions were cold and cheerless, like us. So cold, in fact, that the Coke can on the window ledge next to where Jay slept froze solid.

Feb. 1st: Red alert day! Keith was eligible for a government study involving plasmapheresis. Plasmapheresis is a procedure in which blood is removed from the body, filtered, and returned. The purpose of this filtration is to remove certain proteins from the bloodstream that may be causing the demyelination. If he agreed to participate, we were committed to up to four weeks in "Tundra Land" with the possibility of Keith receiving a sham treatment for two weeks.

The only logical reason I could come up with for entering the study was insurance companies do not currently pay for that treatment with patients with the diagnosis of MS. However, Keith's condition was technically Demyelinating Disease, and I thought there was a good chance his insurance would pay. Even if they did not approve the cost, Keith had enough saved to cover the bill. The obvious advantages of returning to Milwaukee for plasmapheresis were he would receive the authentic treatment initially, and we could be at home. The decision seemed like a simple one to me. The reason Keith even considered the other option was it was presented in such a manner that he felt he would be helping others in similar situations that might not have the savings or insurance to receive the treatment. He was told only if he was an actual participant could his results be used when the decision was made if plasmapheresis was a viable option for people with Multiple Sclerosis. The outcome of that decision would impact insurance companies decisions for payment of the procedure in the future. I really hoped Keith would choose to return to Milwaukee for treatment, however, as a family we had agreed to only support Keith, not try to influence his decisions. This was his battle, and I had my own inner struggles to deal with that day. My proactive type A personality desperately wanted to surface and take control, so it took every ounce of reserve I had to refrain from swaying his decision.

Feb. 1st: (Keith) My speech is so slow and cognitive ability so dull I had to rely on Jason and Mom to ask the questions for me which really makes me feel stupid. I'm thinking about entering a Government Plasmapheresis Research Project whereby I won't know if I'm going to receive the real blood exchange in the first two weeks or second two weeks. If I get significantly better the first two weeks, they will assume I received the actual exchange, and I will be released. The only way I would not get the real treatment is if I got the placebo the first two weeks and get better, but I'd take that too. If I do not show significant improvement, I will stay for another two weeks. At the end of four weeks I will have for sure received the actual treatment. If I agree to this I will need to enter the hospital for up to four weeks. The treatments are in another building, so every other day I will be taken there by ambulance. Mom checked and my insurance will approve physical and occupational therapy while I am in the hospital. This whole experience does not make any sense to me unless I am supposed to go through this to help someone else out. I'm going to pray and think about it before I give the doctor my answer tomorrow. Tonight I'm asking Mom to write down more questions that I have. If I stay, Mom and Jason said they will move into the hospital with me.

Feb. 2nd: Diminished daylight and plummeting temperatures made us feel like even the forces of nature were against us. Every school in the entire state of Minnesota was closed due to the extreme cold. While in Rochester the concept of winter took on a whole new meaning for me. Both illness and winter put me way out of my comfort zone mentally and physically, so I was becoming emotionally brittle. Acutely aware that physical exercise increases my coping ability I had located an indoor pool where I would be able to swim when we registered at the Inn. That morning, just to go swimming, I walked two blocks in the record breaking actual, not wind chill, temperature of 45 degrees below zero thinking I should have my head examined. Yet I knew the very reason I was going was to try to keep from cracking. Before going back out in the dangerous cold I warmed myself and my clothes in the sauna. Therefore, the walk back was refreshing, and I arrived without shivering.

What gave me the cold shivers was in the afternoon when we met for over four hours with the medical team involved in the plasmapheresis project. Within minutes of our scheduled appointment the head of the department briefly joined us. Very matter of factly he informed us that he felt Keith had contracted a rare form of MS, most likely caused by the herpes virus, and he felt even after this episode was under control there was a two-thirds chance it would return sometime during his life. I wonder if doctors have any idea how they can strike unbridled fear in people's hearts with just a few short sentences? He certainly gave no indication that he felt any remorse at having to deliver such disturbing news to us.

Shortly after the doctor made his dooms day proclamation he left, and Keith asked me to go call his insurance case manager for a clarification about payment for continuing physical and occupational therapies if he stayed in Rochester for treatment. What he really wanted was time to discuss with the doctor, with whom the appointment was scheduled, the comment that his problems were caused by the herpes virus. He wanted to know if he caused it himself through sexual activity. According to what he shared with me later, the doctor actually laughed and said absolutely not and then asked Keith if that was why he had sent me out of the room. Keith answered in the affirmative. The neurologist explained that there are numerous types of herpes viruses and the current thought was Keith had been exposed to some form of the virus. Immediately we began asking ourselves where, when, how, and soon discovered on the mountain top, in the chemical plant, and anywhere in between laid the missing piece to the unsolvable puzzle of origin. Now the larger question, looming in front of Keith, was how to treat it without knowing the cause.

At that point Dr. Weinshenker entered the picture. He was the man actually running the plasmapheresis study. For Keith to become an official candidate he was suppose to be completely off steroids, and that is when I intervened. Every time Keith had a reduction of steroids he lost significant cognitive and physical function. I could not fathom stopping his oral steroid medication as a viable option, and tears formed in my eyes as I made my concerns known. That was when I felt the empathy of Dr. Weinshenker and began to build a trust relationship with him, but there was still the whole issue of the placebo possibility. I did not think Keith had the time to risk having the real treatment delayed for two weeks as each day he was getting worse. Plus the thought of him possibly going through seven needless blood filtrations seemed cruel after all he had already been put through. I was becoming more and more convinced the prudent thing to do was to return to Milwaukee.

Keith was hearing the humanitarian aspect of the study. He was buying into the concept of helping others through sacrificially giving of his condition for the benefit of research. I thought of Christ, and realized with a new understanding He truly made the ultimate sacrifice when He offered His body for us. As a mother I did not want Keith to be that sacrificial. I left to telephone his case manager again and was informed his insurance would pay for physical and occupational therapy only. Any additional costs would need to be paid through the research grant or be out of pocket expenses. We then heard some testimonial letters that convinced all of us that plasmapheresis was a viable option. I felt it was the way to go, but I definitely wanted him to go home for treatment. After four hours my knees literally began shaking when Keith said he wanted to participate in the study. I looked him in the eye and told him it was his decision. Jason and I both confirmed we would gladly stay with him. Then I excused myself and went to the bathroom to cry.

Feb. 2nd: (Keith) Interesting day! This morning Jason went with me for a blood draw, and I fainted. Mom was not along which was good news for all of us. Not sure what happened except I started to feel really hot and light headed. I used to feel faint at the sight of needles, but I have been poked so many times in the last months I have gotten used to them. Not really, I've just learned to tolerate needles. I don't think anyone could ever get used to them. Decided to enter the study. The way I see it, if I don't participate the doctors here will just have a casual interest in me and my case whereas if I enter the study, I believe they will take an active interest in me which will help me in the long run. Plus, if plasmapheresis works there may be another time I will need it, and then I will have a convincing case for my insurance to pay for a second round of treatments. I can see how this might help others, and the only thing it is costing me is time. I am not doing anything else productive with my time right now, so I might as well try to help others as well as myself at this point in my life.

Feb. 3rd: Woke up to numbing cold. This was the first winter with my car and Jason tried to start it the way the other car always started, which was a huge mistake. By the time I thought to check the owner's manual to discover the correct and different procedure, the battery had little life and simply sputtered "in your dreams." The topic of discussion in the largest patient waiting rooms I have ever seen was how many cars started in the various hotel parking lots. Unfortunately, our car had now joined the silent majority. We were literally part of history as Rochester was recording its coldest temperatures ever. Fred's cousin, Jim, had invited us for dinner, and fortunately offered us a ride, for when I called for a jump start the wait was eight hours, which confirmed how paralyzing those frigid temperatures were.

Being able to spend a few hours in a comfortably warm house was wonderful, and we enjoyed good home cooking while listening to some of the youthful adventures of Fred and his cousin. Our favorite story was when Fred's cousin described an era when all their mutual friends thought it was "cool" to figure out how to make their cars look and go fast. Everyone, that is, except conservative Fred who was busy installing seat belts in his 1956 Chevy. On the way back to the hotel we all agreed as much fun as it was to have a "Fred Roast," it would have been even better if he could have been there to give his versions of the stories. Once back, the three of us worked on the first official issue of the Kelroy Gazette.

Kelroy Gazette

Volume 1 Issue 1 **February 2, 1996**

UPDATE ON KEITH

Maybe Mayo Until March

The neurologists at the Mayo Clinic are now hypothesizing that Keith's demylination is being caused by an unidentified virus. According to the doctors, this does not, however, conclusively rule out the existence, or the future existence, of Multiple Sclerosis.

The next recommended treatment for Keith is a process called plasma pherosis. Keith has agreed to receive this treatment as part of a government study taking place at the Mayo. This will involve a two to four week stay in Rochester, depending on whether Keith receives the placebo or actual treatment during the first two weeks. In the event that Keith does not show a moderate to marked improvement in two weeks, he will then be crossed over to the other treatment, thus assuring him the actual treatment.

Karen and Jason are currently the ones staying in Rochester with Keith. Karen is planning on staying for at least one more week and Jason will be with Keith throughout his treatment. As of Wednesday, they will all be staying at St. Mary's Hospital, with Keith in the GNRC Unit and Karen and Jason in the Guest Accommodations Center.

We are all asking for your continued prayers as Keith begins this next procedure. Please pray that he may receive the actual treatment first and have a positive response, thus allowing us all to return to Racine as early as possible. In addition to prayers, letters and phone calls would also be very much appreciated.

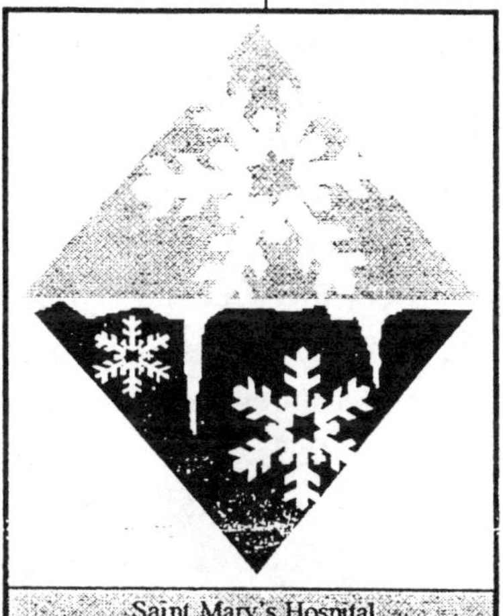

Saint Mary's Hospital
1216 2nd St. SW
Rochester, MN 55902

Keith Kelroy
GNRC Unit
(507) 255-5123

Jason Kelroy
Guest Accommodations
(507) 255-5581

OTHER NEWS

The Silver Lining

Jason received some great news in the mail yesterday and once again proved that every cloud has a silver lining. His first semester law grades arrived and we were all ecstatic to find out that, despite the extra-stress of his brother's illness, he had earned an "A" average, which places him in the top 20% of his law school classmates. He would like to thank everyone who kept him in their prayers over the past semester. Keith seems to be a little bit worried, however, that perhaps the miracle went to the wrong family member. He asks that everyone please "re-confirm" their requests with the Lord.

Moving on from our "hot" family news, the weather here in Rochester is absolutely frigid (-35). In fact, it was so cold across the entire state that the governor closed all of the state schools. And the can of soda that we kept by our window has frozen solid. Unfortunately for Jason, that is the very same window that he gets to sleep by. We are all trying our best to keep warm. It's not easy!

WHEN SENDING MAIL TO KEITH OR JASON: Please make sure to put the appropriate person and unit (GNRC or Guest Accommodations) on the envelope.

Top Five Minnesota State Slogans	
1	MN - closed for glacial repairs!
2	Jump start your car lately?
3	Many are cold but few are frozen!
4	Minnesota - glove it or leave it!
5	Our visitors all turn blue(with envy)!

CHAPTER NINE

St. Mary's Hospital - Rochester, Minnesota

Feb. 4th: In the morning I started to walk to a church that Fred's cousin told me about, but soon succumbed to the frigid temperature and sought warmth in the first church I came upon, which I discovered was the oldest church in Rochester. Their service did not begin for another half hour, so I passed the time in the church library. The only book I happened to remove from the shelves was about a young woman who had died at age 23. I cannot remember the title of the book or what initially attracted me to it, but it was another "God sighting" because the message confirmed my belief that what I wanted most for my children was eternal salvation which was not dependent on reaching a ripe old age. I found comfort in the book and the service. After church, I hurried back, collected the guys, and drove to the local discount center to stock up on the items we would need for our extended stay.

Keith was always a saver and believed generic was the only brand on the market. Once in the health and beauty section he found a huge bottle of generic shampoo for 89 cents that he thought would be perfect. The only thing that would have made it better was if it had been on sale. I had successfully taught him to look for sales, but for him generic was the ultimate discovery of how to save money without worrying about sales or coupons. Keith was a buyer not a shopper. He would enter a store to make a purchase only when absolutely necessary. Jason and I unsuccessfully tried to talk him out of purchasing the shampoo. Following shopping we stopped for lunch at Boston Chicken.

The previous May Boston Chicken had catered Jason's college graduation party. It was a lawn party held on an absolutely perfect spring day where over 120 people gathered to celebrate with us. We had set up a Dells Frozen Lemonade Stand where people congregated to exchange the news. It was fun reliving the memories of that special day. Jason had been on the UW homecoming court in his junior year. The court was brought on the Camp Randall football field in the Bucky Wagon which was an old time firetruck. For his party our neighbor had located an antique fire engine and owner who willingly brought it to our house for the start of the party. We took Jason's picture with every guest in front of the engine. At the time when our neighbor realized we hadn't had our picture taken and asked us to gather at the truck, I was hesitant because the food had just arrived. I am grateful for her persistence because it turned out to be our last family picture before Keith got sick.

Following lunch we admitted Keith to the hospital, his third St. Mary's. That night Jason stayed with Keith in his hospital room. I spent the night in a lonely hotel room, far from home, with only the company of memories of happier times to help me fall asleep.

Feb. 4th: (Keith) Here we go again. I'm on the fifth floor of the largest hospital I have ever seen. I refused the wheelchair and insisted on walking to my room which was not the smartest thing because by the time I got here I was limping, tired, and

Mom gave me no sympathy. Later, I asked my nurse how far it was to the admitting desk, and she estimated a half mile. She also told me this place has 18 miles of corridors. The wing I am on is entirely set up for research. Pretty scary to come to Mayo's for answers and the best they can do is put me in an experimental program. I may need to heal myself, but I am going to get better.

Feb. 5th: Moving day again! This time Jason and I admitted ourselves to the hospital. When I told my friends that, they teasingly responded, "sounds serious." This St. Mary's was located a mile from the Colonial Inn, and Jay and I decided we wanted to be closer to Keith. At the time Keith agreed to enter the study Dr. Weinshenker's nurse told us about a wing on one of the many floors of the hospital that outpatients and family members could rent on a nightly basis. The concept was popular, and a room first became available on this date. The only differences between our wing and Keith's was one room had been converted into a laundry room and there was a little kitchen for guests to use. Our beds were hospital beds, fully equipped with all the buttons for positioning and operating the radio and television. It looked just like a regular hospital room and had that same antiseptic aroma. We had to adjust to hearing "Code Red" with a room location which was usually followed by "All Clear" a couple of times during the night and the whir of helicopters as the Flight for Life Helicopter landed just outside our window. The biggest adjustment was for Jason and me to learn to share limited space. I tend to like things orderly while he is most comfortable in an environment that can best be described as organized chaos. Ask him for anything and he knows exactly where it is among the disarray. Therefore, we recognized we needed to honor each others space, but agreed a safe path through to my half of the room was a reasonable request.

Jason enjoyed lounging so found it comfortable to move between rooms in his flannel pants, T-shirt, and slippers while Keith preferred his basketball shorts, T-shirt, and socks. Consequently, Jason often appeared to be the patient when he was in Keith's room. Staying in the hospital provided the wonderful advantage of 24 hour access to Keith without going out in the cold. We would leave Keith's room sometime around ten at night, and one of us would be back down there when he woke in the morning. On treatment days that meant Jason was there by seven in the morning. On non-treatment days Keith would get up around nine, and I would be there. Keith never was a loner, so he always preferred to have one of us with him. Fortunately, we all enjoyed being with each other.

Feb 5th: (Keith) I'm in a double room, and tonight my first official roommate arrived. Last night Jason slept over. I don't like the idea of sharing a room with a stranger. How stupid to even have double rooms. At least I am mobile and well

Feb. 6th: Jason went with Keith for his first plasmapheresis treatment. The procedure was done in the Hilton building which was across from the Colonial Inn where we previously stayed. For all 14 trips Keith was transported there by ambulance. The actual procedure was done in a large room that contained eight hospital beds surrounding a nurses' station. Each bed had its own bank of machinery to treat blood disorders.

Once Keith was wheeled in he was moved from his cart to the bed. Then IV lines were hooked up to each arm and the filtration process began. The blood was drawn out of one arm, run through the filter machine and then pumped back into his other arm. His entire blood was cycled through the machinery several times each treatment which took a couple of hours. During that time whoever was with Keith would visit with him, watch a video, or sleep. Riding in an ambulance to watch Keith's blood being filtered was something I preferred not to do, and Jason said he didn't mind going, especially if he could use the siren.

The first day while they were gone I went swimming. The walk to the pool was a little more than a mile, so I was relieved it had warmed up, it almost reached zero. Afterwards I walked downtown to pick up a newspaper and the best chocolate chip muffin I have ever eaten. I returned to the hospital just as they arrived back in Keith's room. They were in amazingly good spirits and joked about how they tried to talk the ambulance driver into taking them through McDonald's drive through. Jason went to our room, and I spent the next several hours with Keith reading the paper and mail, eating lunch, and losing at Scrabble. While we were playing in the lounge we had the opportunity to meet a grandfather, named Stan, who was alone at the hospital for a three week stay while receiving experimental treatment for a rare eye disease. Stan enjoyed playing Scrabble thus we adopted him as an honorary member of our family. The first time he played with us he used all seven of his tiles to make the word "mudders" which we learned are horses that run well in the mud. He was obviously a good player and over the next few weeks many hours were spent in healthy competition.

When Keith went to physical and occupational therapy, Jason and I switched places. Usually I would then spend some time in the chapel. This chapel was the size of a large church. I would often just sit in silence letting my thoughts flow freely. There was one picture of Christ wearing His crown of thorns that consistently caught and held my attention. Eventually I realized what captivated me was the artist had depicted Christ's eyes just as sad as Keith's.

Late afternoons and evenings we spent as a threesome, and each night before going to sleep Jason and I would play a game of Cribbage which gave us an opportunity to interact with each other. We shared worrisome thoughts we never mentioned to Keith, and I often wondered how many of those same thoughts Keith kept to himself. We always tried to be positively positive around Keith which mirrored the image he portrayed to us. Individually I guess we decided to squeeze happiness from each day. Therefore, I lived life on the surface, not probing deeper to figure it all out. Knowing Keith was not in physical pain, a good game of Scrabble, drinking a cold Diet Coke, hearing the words "I love you Mom" from my sons, and Fred's voice on the phone made for many good days during bad times.

Feb. 6th: (Keith) Hopefully I've completed one of seven treatments instead of one of 14. Really wasn't a bad experience. I was taken by ambulance from St. Mary's to a building called the Hilton. The room had eight beds and mine was the only one with the machines covered in sheets, so we would not know if I was receiving the real or sham treatment. We asked how we would be able to tell if I was receiving the real treatment or a placebo, and the technician said by the speed at which the filter was set. I had an IV in each arm. One took the blood out, and then it was filtered and pumped back through the other IV. The whole thing took about two hours, and I slept some of the time. Before this is over I'll look like a druggie with all the needle marks in my arms.

Feb. 8th: The morning was a repeat of his first treatment, except that Keith was exhausted from not being able to sleep the night before due to his roommate's snoring. Jason had successfully lobbied for Keith to be moved to a private room. That afternoon Jason left to spend the weekend in Madison. Keith had offered to pay Jason's rent which was appreciated because Jason was under a year's lease. We felt Jason made a huge sacrifice to put his education on hold, and did not want him to also give up his entire social life, especially since Carrie was waiting for him in Madison. Carrie and Jason had started dating in high school, so deciding to leave her and law school in Madison was a monumental decision. When he left I felt a sense of abandonment and began to appreciate just how long that week in January had been for Fred. With the exception of one cousin in the area, Keith and I were now physically alone. We had met several patients who were really here alone because their families could not afford to join them, and we thought how difficult that must be. Fortunately, the phone rang continuously that night.

Feb. 8th: (Keith) I would never make it in a double room. I told them today to bill me, but please find me a private room. I was kept awake most of last night by my roommate. Fortunately, a room opened up unexpectantly, and they said I could have it for three days. Mom spent the afternoon decorating the room by hanging up the many cards I have already received with surgical tape. When I asked if she should be taping on the walls she smiled and told me no one had asked for a security deposit. She thinks if the room looks decorated they might not have the heart to move me which would be great because this room is perfect. It is large and is actually set off from the hallway by a double entrance so it is really quiet. No dramatic improvement. That's about it.

Feb. 9th: Fred arrived, and we went out for dinner which was a mistake. We had to wait for a table in the bar area which was packed full of people Keith's age just out for a normal, fun, youthful Friday night. Keith became very quiet and withdrawn. It was obvious Jason's presence was missed because he could always make Keith laugh while distracting him from fully taking in the big picture.

Feb. 9th: (Keith) Have been here at Mayo's for over a week. My speech is worse from last week. My vision has definitely worsened, and there is some dizziness with the vision. Other things have held relatively constant. Today was a hard day. I am working at keeping a good attitude, would like to see someone who can do better. I am going to hang in there and fight this thing to the end. Good night!

Feb. 10th: Surviving this extended hospital stay meant escaping from it regularly. We saw every movie that was in Rochester the six weeks we were there. Often we would separate at the popcorn stand with the men taking in the action films while I headed for the relaxing romantics. We all enjoyed the comedies and those contrived humorous situations were welcome reprieves from the seriousness of our real world. One huge indication that we were in a city controlled by the medical world was when we saw people in the theaters and shopping center wearing bathrobes.

Feb. 10th: (Keith) Dad went to treatment with me. We were the only ones there this morning and Dad said it reminded him of the Wizard of Oz with the mystery machines hid behind sheets. The technician offered Dad a bed, and we both slept during the treatment. Later went to the movie and out for supper. At dinner I told Mom and Dad if I never get better than I am right now, I would still be glad to be alive, but this is as low as I can imagine going and still feel life is worth living. It was a pretty good day. Some enjoyment out of life.

Feb. 11th: Jason returned in time for brunch so we could celebrate Fred's birthday. When Jason saw Keith he suggested he wash his hair informing him it was really looking greasy. Keith replied he had washed it that morning, and then figured out why the shampoo he bought was only 89 cents. We were quick to point out to Keith sometimes you get exactly what you pay for. Jason went and got his own shampoo bottle, and Keith rewashed his hair while Fred opened his gifts. We had hoped and prayed to be able to give Fred the gift of seeing significant improvement in Keith, but Fred received no such present. However, he was enjoying the gift of presence. The guys were both in good moods and entertained us with their wit and phenomenal attitudes. Keith was concerned he wasn't talking clearly, to which Jason replied that sometimes happens after a Saturday night. I could only detect a slight lisp.

It is tradition, in our family, to reflect on your birthday the three best and worst happenings of the year. For best Fred selected our family vacation to Lake Tahoe, Jason receiving his acceptance into law school, and Keith moving to Madison. For worst it was the initial drive to Madison after I called to tell him something was seriously wrong with Keith, the day of his surgery, and the January trip to Mayo's. Following dessert Fred began the long lonely drive home without the gift he valued most, his family.

Feb. 14th: Valentines Day and for the first time in years I was dateless. We spent the evening at Fred's cousin's home. Following a delicious dinner we didn't have to order off a menu Barb and I became engaged in a discussion about the futility of worry. I shared of all the countless things I worried about while raising the guys, Demyelinating Disease was not one of them. She told me her wise grandfather often commented it doesn't pay to worry because the real problems in life will sneak up on your backside. Within hours of our conversation she received a call her father had died unexpectedly which was a strong reminder my worry time would be better spent in prayer time.

Feb. 14th: (Keith) Today was another good day on the new scale of good and bad days. Emotionally a good day. I had a nurse say to me, "Be realistic." No! I refuse to be realistic. If I am realistic, I will not recover 100%. I am too damn stubborn to be realistic. There are times when I feel like I want to quit, pout, and whatever. But no, not tonight. Tonight I want to beat this thing, and I am going to beat this thing no matter how long it takes. That is how I feel tonight. And another thing, as long as I am alive I will keep fighting.

Feb. 15th: When Fred saw me over the weekend he was very concerned about my weight loss and indicated he was not comfortable with me staying in Rochester for the second round of treatments. I was frustrated by his position because I had initially told Fred that Jason and I would remain at Rochester as long as Keith was there. I was emotionally doing okay, and had even developed a close enough relationship with the nursing staff that they showed me where the key to unlock the refrigerator was hidden, so I would always have access to Diet Coke. The only significant problem was my loss of appetite which was something I could not control.

Food did not look, smell, or taste good, and what I did eat felt horrible once consumed. As long as I didn't eat I was fine so that was how I elected to solve the food dilemma. My main concern was most of my clothes were no longer fitting whereas Fred was worried about my actual lack of weight and wanted to get me home and back to school. He said he had enough to worry about without adding me to his list, and I felt like I was letting him down.

I certainly wasn't trying to lose weight for attention and actually resented it when anyone pointed it out to me. I think people have different responses to stress, but I do believe there are physical consequences to prolonged stress. That is why I faithfully did something outdoors and physical everyday and why I wanted Keith to have physical therapy each day. As far as my staying in Rochester the guys did not seem to care which one of us was with them, in fact both of them independently shared with me they wanted either Fred or me with them but it made no difference which one. I spent part of the day trying to write a letter to be sent to our family and friends updating them about Keith and our new projected plan of action. It was difficult to communicate that information because I felt like a failure.

Feb. 15th (Keith) Pretty good day. Saw a little bit of improvement. Real slow. My doctors were in, and it looks like I am going to be here another two weeks as of Sunday. I don't know how I feel about that. At least that way I am assured of the real treatment. We won't wonder, we'll know. I am going to hang in there. I feel upbeat tonight, ready to take on tomorrow. I really feel like I am going to beat this thing, Two years, two months, it is a short segment out of my relatively short life and I just need to keep telling myself that, although it seems unbearably long now that I am going to get through it, I will look back on it and I will say gosh I made it through that, I can make it through anything.

Feb. 17th: My brother Fred had driven up from Kansas City and Jason and I headed for home. My brother said he was comfortable flying solo with Keith for the weekend. As we left Rochester heading east, they headed south to scout out our dad's boyhood home in Leroy, Minnesota. I dropped Jason off in Madison on my way to Racine. It was wonderful to see Fred waiting at the door for me, and I admitted to myself a part of me was very relieved to be home.

Feb. 18: Staying home would have been ideal but selfish as there was a surprise 80th birthday party for Fred's stepmother in Fond du Lac. As often as Fred's parents had been there for us, those past months, we wanted to make the effort to be physically present on her special day. From our new perspective reaching 80 was a monumental accomplishment and something worth celebrating. It was a difficult day because everyone was concerned about Keith, and kept asking us the same questions. It would have been easier, but not appropriate, to make just one public announcement. Appreciating their concern, and needing everyone's support made us vulnerable as we were now living a pretty public life, while dealing with such complex personal matters.

Feb. 18th: (Keith) I am having some speech problems. Tomorrow is the day when the doctors decide if I have to go another fourteen days on this treatment. I hope I got the placebo because if I didn't it means that the treatment didn't work, and I will have to get better on my own. I am pretty confident that the doctors are going to tell me that I have not improved dramatically. I am certain I have gotten the placebo. Today was a real good day. My uncle, Fred, from Kansas City was up here. Probably walked the most I have since Christmas. I continue to decrease my Prednisone dosage. The demyelination seems to have moved primarily to my face and arm. The face and arm are right next to each other in the brain. I just hope there is not significant myelin damage.

Feb. 19th: Fred and I exchanged emotional good-byes as he left for Rochester when I left for school. Within minutes of my arrival I discovered all my student files were missing from my computer. Fortunately, before I became completely hysterical our competent computer aide located them in my hard drive. I have an unusual computer in the sense it can act as two computers, and somehow all my records had been transferred within the hard drive to the second computer without leaving a visual prompt on my screen. Being totally consumed with that current crisis I was able to temporarily and successfully separate myself from worrying about what was happening with Keith. At the end of that hectic day I knew it still felt good to be back. I am fortunate that I not only care about my students but they also care about me. Many of the cards hanging in Keith's room were made for him by my students. On the wall by my desk I have an 11x14 picture of our family. Even before Keith got sick the kids frequently asked me questions about my family, but now their questions increased in frequency and intensity.

Feb. 19th: (Keith) It's official. I will be here another 14 days. Dad arrived for round two. Also found out today I was accepted into Business School at the University of Wisconsin. I'm still not sure if I will go to school or return to work. Right now it looks like I will go for my MBA. If I do Jason and I plan on sharing an apartment with his friend. Jason just found out he made the Dean's List first semester, and I'm really proud of him. I told him I expect us both in school next semester, but he is to go for sure or I'll kick his butt.

Feb. 20th: (Keith) I started the second round of treatments today. I will be here for another two weeks. If I didn't get the placebo I am still going to get better. I just have this feeling. The doctors don't really know what this is, they just keep saying severe demyelination. There is no mechanism to look at myelin yet, but they know that myelin does have the potential to repair itself. I am going to have to settle in for another two weeks. Today was a hard day, realizing it will be another two long weeks. Today will probably be the hardest day of the second two weeks, I hope. I have faith and confidence that I am going to get better and I will be in school come fall. As it goes on, it does get harder to keep my faith and my attitude, but I am doing well. I would like to see someone who could do better. I am going to hang in there and fight this thing to the end. Good night.

Feb. 24th: (Keith) I had my third treatment, and I am seeing signs of improvement. My speech has cleared up. Three days ago it was absolutely horrible and I knew it. I am cognitively alert. My right hand is opening more, and my right foot is moving more. Nothing too drastic, but definitely in the right direction. Hopefully the doctors will be as impressed as I am when they come in tomorrow. I am looking forward to seeing the doctors' reactions. I am confident in saying the plaque is no longer growing. We have halted it.

Feb. 25th: I did not drive up to Rochester for the weekend. I knew Penny and Vern were leaving from Madison on Friday and taking my mom. Their daughter Julie was also coming from Luther College in Decorah, Iowa. In addition Fred's parents were arriving Sunday and spending the night. Instead I went to early church which was still a comfortable place for me. I did not understand what was happening to Keith, but was at some spiritual peace with the situation. I was becoming more and more convinced Keith belonged to God, and that we were just given the wonderful privilege of raising him. My panicked based petitions had stopped, and my prayer was now simply, very simply "Thy will be done."

Following service I met Ginny at Lakeside Mall which is half way between Naperville and Racine. For a few brief hours life seemed normal and normal felt magnificent. It bothers me to pay full price for clothes, so I was pleased when I found a simple tailored black dress on sale that I knew would be a perfect wardrobe staple. I envisioned wearing it on a number of occasions as I was hopeful about being able to resurrect my social life in the not too distant future. I cheerfully wrote out the check focusing on what I was saving instead of what I was spending. When I purchase clothes I mentally divide the cost of the article by the anticipated number of wearings, and this time I had located a real bargain. Ironically, I only wore the dress once.

Feb. 25th: (Keith) Probably my best day since I've been up here for the last month and a half. Cognitively I woke up this morning feeling different. I felt cognitively much sharper. My speech is immensely better. My hand is starting to open slightly more. My foot is moving up. I could always make it go down, but not up and now I am starting to do that. I feel different than I did the last two weeks after treatment. I feel real lethargic, light headed, and faint after I receive the treatment which lasts for about half a day. In fact today I actually fainted right after the treatment. The first two weeks I had none of those symptoms. I think those are all good signs that I am getting the real treatment. I know I am going to recover 100%, it is just a feeling I have. The doctors were pleasantly surprised at how my speech and movement have progressed. Things are going in the right direction. Now we just have to wait. I'll have an MRI Friday or Monday and see if it confirms what I feel. Then I don't know if they will do anything more. Most likely it will just be a lot of waiting and a lot of patience, but I can do it.

Feb. 27th: (Keith) Once again I have improved over the night. I am stronger. In therapy I could climb the hand ladder. Five days ago I could not get to the first peg. Today I could get all the way up. I also could ride a stationary bike. I'm noticing a lot of improvement that has to be due to the swelling going down. I wore jeans for the first time in a month. Cognitively I feel sharp. I feel really good. I am on top of the world tonight. I am going to beat this thing. I go home next Monday. I will only be on 10mg of Prednisone starting tomorrow. That's about it.

Feb. 28th: With the daily positive news reports coming from Rochester I was doing quite well. It was the first time in my life I lived alone for any length of time. Many people offered to come stay with me, but I really enjoyed being responsible only for myself and the dog. I caught up at school, lingered in the bathtub, and played my classical music as loud as I wanted. Fred likes rock and roll, particularly Elvis, so we have an understanding his music is on his time and my music is on my time. I also completed reading C.S. Lewis' book <u>Mere Christianity</u>. It was a period of time where I went inward for strength and centered myself. I see God in the acts of others, but I find God in the depths of my soul.

To handle any crisis I need time and space to meditate, reflect, and refocus. I discovered two main things about myself during those weeks. First I realized I was becoming more comfortable with my personal relationship with God. One night when I was with Keith, Fred had met with our small church group and they had watched a video about the apostle John. Fred said he thought I might like to see it, so it was sitting on the television when I came home. While watching the video it occurred to me that none of the apostles had an easy life, for them to say yes to Christ was to say yes to suffering. The significant comfort I gleaned from that realization was the idea that maybe what we were going through was not because God was mad at us or didn't care about us, perhaps the meaning in all this was the direct opposite; for some unknown reason He personally chose us to witness for Him. I pondered that realizing if it was true what we were going through was meaningful instead of meaningless. "We" is the correct word because I was truly amazed how often Keith used the word we when describing something that he was going through. He obviously viewed this as a family illness, and so did we.

The second thing I discovered was my relationship with doctors was dependent on their message. Those who delivered hope like Dr. Cameron, who felt there was a chance this was not Multiple Sclerosis, and Dr. Weinshenker who honestly believed plasmapheresis had the potential to help Keith I could relate to. Doctors who reported Keith was experiencing, "severe fulminating Multiple Sclerosis" I could not identify with. There is nothing hopeful about the words Atypical Fulminant Multiple Sclerosis. Atypical meant Keith had something of unknown origin with a small knowledge base from which to learn about it, Fulminant meant explosive and unpredictable, and Multiple Sclerosis meant incurable where determination would not be enough to overcome the devastation of the disease. Keith's type of MS was a cruel disease because it continually assaulted him without warning or reason. He never had any prolonged chance to make the necessary modifications so he could get on with his life, because just when he did, it returned for another attack. Consequently, every time a doctor spoke of any of those words they took our hope away and therefore I did not want to believe them because for us to survive we needed to keep our faith and hope. Often the message and the manner in which it was delivered determined my relationship with the messenger.

CHAPTER TEN

St. Mary's Hospital - Racine, Wisconsin

Feb. 29th: (Keith) I am really tired tonight. Otherwise I am feeling great. I can't believe how much better I've gotten. It really is a miracle. This treatment is working better than anybody hoped. The doctors were in to see me today, and they referred to what they saw as dramatic improvement. I will be out of here on Tuesday. That's about it. I don't feel much like talking, but that in no way reflects how I am doing. Overall, I couldn't ask for more progress or a better recovery.

March 2nd: Fred arrived home looking much better than the last time he came from Rochester. We both agreed we couldn't have done it without Jason. Except for weekends, Jason had been up in Rochester with Keith the entire time. Keith was extremely fortunate to have him for his best friend, and we are blessed to have him as our son. Jason wasn't too excited that Fred was leaving, but Keith was going to be released Sunday and would move in with Jason for two nights until all his out-patient tests and appointments were completed. The room was not big enough for three and no one liked the idea of packing up and moving again, so Fred decided to move out. Keith had kept his oversized private fully decorated room for most of his stay at Mayo's, and the staff said they never had a patient receive more mail. By the time he had to transfer to a smaller room, for the last few days, all four walls were filled with cards, banners, and messages of cheer. We were now in our sixth month, and people were still interacting in our lives on a daily basis in large numbers. Fred indicated he would need to live to a ripe old age just to pay people back for all the acts of kindness bestowed on us.

With Jason bringing Keith home, Fred and I would both be able to work a full week for the first time in months. Going through something of this magnitude changed our entire lifestyle. Our hectic happy life before Keith got sick had become a distant memory, and it seemed like we had all the time in the world for him because nothing else mattered. I originally began calling it the season of stress, then when it went on longer I referred to it as the season of cancellations, and by now we had all stepped out of the fast lane for what turned out to be the year of the zebra. Our only consistent outside activities were school and church.

That night we went to church, and when we got home Jason was on the phone. Keith was concerned because his lip was starting to tingle, and Jason wished we were there. We talked to Keith and encouraged him to try and focus on an activity instead of his body. They called back a few hours later, said they were both doing fine and the tingling had gone away. We knew that both Keith and Jason looked to us for assurance and it was important we continued to demonstrate hope and confidence everything would turn out fine.

March 3rd: (Keith) I have completed four weeks of treatments. I have seen some pretty miraculous results. Dad has gone home, and Jason and I will follow shortly.

Now all I need is to get off the Prednisone real slowly. It feels really good to be leaving the hospital. I just hope the progress continues. I think it is going to, I know it is going to continue. I think I am going to be in school come September.

March 5th: The guys arrived home, and it was wonderful to all be together again. We functioned much better as a foursome. Many friends came over and what I expected to be a quiet arrival ended up a party. A celebration punctuated with crescendos of laughter interspersed amidst the constant conversation. Balloons, presents, and homemade treats also marked the occasion. The gifts that intrigued me the most were two wooden name plaques. One said "Jason-Healer" and the other "Keith-God's Warrior." I thought they were specially made but was told they weren't which surprised me considering how fitting the descriptions were. It was a wonderful homecoming wrapped in love and friendship. It was good to once again have our home filled with people and the sounds of laughter. Our dog, Sam, wagged his tail the entire night as he moved from person to person and if I had one I would have been happily wagging mine also.

March 5th: (Keith) Jason and I have left St. Mary's. We are in the car heading home. I have been up here five weeks and I don't know if I will recognize my home. Things are going real good. The doctors explained to me about the MRI being less enhanced. I asked what that meant in laymen's terms and was told it's the greatest indicator of how active the disease is and so they are assuming my disease is no longer active. They don't know how long it will last, but I am going to assume forever. I need to go back to Mayo's in a month, but we're out of here. Over and out.

March 7th: (Keith) I continue to feel good. My hand is opening up a little more each day. I'm beginning to not wear out as quick. My stamina is increasing. I made plans to go see Phil on March 30th, and I'm going to be in good shape that weekend. He really hasn't seen me in good shape, but I am going to be that weekend. Previously every time he has come up, or I've gone down, I've deteriorated, but that is not going to happen this time. I feel different this time. I feel like I've hit the end of the road. I know I've said that before, but this time there is a different feeling. Now I need to focus on the day to day and not look at the big picture. I can't think about how much I have to get back. Six months, two years, whatever it takes I'll have it all back. Then I'll look back and think I made it through this. That is how I feel today.

March 10th: (Keith) Found out today I qualify to receive Social Security benefits. I am surprised because when I went to fill out the forms I was told it was a for-

mality to activate my Long Term Disability Insurance and 90% of the claims are rejected the first time. Therefore, it is not reassuring to think the government doesn't believe I can return to my job, but then seldom does the government make fiscally responsible decisions. If I do decide to return to school, it certainly makes it much more affordable.

March 11th: Fred had afternoon and evening school conferences so did not need to leave for work until after ten. The last thing he did before leaving at 10:15 a.m. was go downstairs and say good-bye to Keith. He found him resting comfortably on the couch. At 10:30 a.m. I was notified I had an important call. I had just begun administrating the state third grade reading test, so knew something was terribly wrong for me to be called out of class. Jason was on the phone. He was speaking so fast I had a difficult time understanding what he was telling me. He kept saying Keith was acting very strange and not making any sense. I could not exactly comprehend what Jason was trying to describe so told him to try and slow down and calmly explain what was happening. He kept repeating Keith was saying and doing things that weren't right and he was scared. I asked where they were and Jason said downstairs, and he kept reiterating Keith was not cooperating with him. In fact he said Keith was acting like he wanted to hurt him. I could tell by the tone of Jason's voice he was really uncomfortable being alone with Keith so I told him to hang up, dial 911, and I would meet them at the hospital. I called Fred before he even had time to arrive at school and told his secretary to have him meet us at the hospital. By the time the ambulance arrived Jason had been able to get Keith upstairs. Keith was still pretty uncooperative, but now Jason had some support. While Keith could not communicate verbally, he physically insisted on changing his clothes before he'd agree to go the hospital. This would be Keith's fourth St. Mary's Hospital. By the time I arrived, at St. Mary's, it was determined Keith had experienced a focal seizure. Keith was beginning to verbally respond and was angry at the nurse who tried to put an I.D. bracelet on him. I promised him he would not have to stay overnight, as we both looked at each other with tears in our eyes. I silently petitioned God to let my words be true. Six weeks at Mayo's for six good days did not seem right.

Within minutes Fred arrived at the hospital. Keith was now able to speak coherently again, and he kept asking us if he was making sense. He explained that previously when Jason could not understand what he was saying he thought he was talking just as rationally as he was now. In his mind he had no understanding of why Jason was not comprehending what he was saying and it really made him mad. At the time Keith was aware something was wrong, but it appeared Jason was not helping him. Jason was still visibly upset, so we encouraged him to go home. The three of us were released within three hours following a cat-scan and an intravenous dose of Dilantin.

That night Jason was more upset than Keith. He said it was a terrible experience, and that he had never been so scared. Jason was a housefellow at a Madison dorm for two years and had dealt with many unpleasant things so I was amazed the seizure went right to the top of his list of never to be repeated experiences. As a housefellow he was directly responsible for about 60 students in the dorm and indirectly for the entire student population of the building. Over the years Jason has had to call 911 on numerous occasions. Yet there was something unique about this emergency, and it totally unnerved him. Keith seemed to take it all in stride and appeared most upset about not being able to have a beer at his fraternity's annual Beach Party.

March 12th: (Keith) March 11th was an interesting day. I had a seizure. Unbeknownst to me, I went to sleep and had a seizure. I woke up still on the couch, but I couldn't talk. My speech was completely gone. When I came out of my seizure I was yelling upstairs to my brother. He couldn't understand what I was saying, but I thought I was making perfect sense. I wasn't as it was all garbled speech. Jason gave me paper to write what I was saying. I couldn't write either. When he showed me afterwards what I wrote, I don't blame him for not being able to figure out what I was saying. I just wrote letters like X,Y,P,and Z, but at the time I was really mad at him because I thought I was writing him a perfectly clear message. At one point I even picked up a chair and wanted to throw it at him. I did end up going to the Emergency Room via ambulance. By the time we got to the hospital my speech was starting to come back and some arm movement. My fine motor coordination came back gradually, and tonight I am talking pretty much normal. My Dilantin level was 5.3 where previously it had been between 9 and 11. The therapeutic level is between 10 and 20. The doctors at Mayo decided I could go off Dilantin because I did not think I ever had a seizure before, but come to find out during the LSAT exam I probably had one. I had a headache two or three days in advance of the exam just like the one I've had for the past two days. It got really sharp when I shook my head back and forth just like the one last September. So when I couldn't remember the instructor giving the directions, I most likely had a seizure during that time. The good thing is I had a warning sign, and I don't think there is any permanent damage from the seizure. The bad news is I'm now going to have to stay on Dilantin for one to two years which means no beer at Beach Party, or the next Beach Party, but that's fine I'll have a good time anyways. Okay!

March 16th: Jason had gone to Madison to see Carrie. He called to tell us he was an emotional wreck. At first I thought something had happened between the two of them, but he shared he was just having a horrible time getting over Keith's seizure and indicated if at all possible he would appreciate being away from home a few more days. By now Fred was on the other line and we suggested Jason stay in Madison until it felt comfortable for him to come home, and suggested perhaps he might want to talk to a counselor. He indicated he knew a counselor from his house-fellow days, and thought he would give her a call. I called my mom, who was our ever ready back-up, and she gladly agreed to come.

CHAPTER ELEVEN

Sacred Heart Rehabilitation Hospital - Milwaukee, Wisconsin

March 17th: (Keith) St. Patty's Day! Went to Fond du Lac to celebrate with the family. Had a good time tipping some O'Douls with my relatives. Today I noticed my right ankle could move in a circular direction for the first time in over two months. The doctors at Mayo's said they feared there was permanent nerve damage to the right foot, but there was no way to tell for sure and I would just have to wait and see. If function returned then there was no permanent damage, if not there was permanent damage. It came back. Things are going real well right now. My biggest problem is screwing around trying to get my Dilantin level adjusted. The body can change how it metabolizes the medicine which affects the metabolic rate and the effectiveness of the dose. The doctors are erring on the high side but hopefully in four days things will level out. I have to stay at a level for five days to get an accurate reading. I'm sure I'm too high now because I'm experiencing a little bit of confusion. Sacred Heart put off cognitive testing until next week. Good-night!

March 18th: (Keith) I feel different. There is an aura that I have never felt before going through my body. I really can't explain it. The disease is going away. Whatever it is, it is leaving. I'm just so happy it's going away. I keep putting my trust in God.

March 20th: (Keith) I continue to do very well. My toes are moving, and my gait is a lot better. I continue to wean off my Prednisone, and the doctors are still working at obtaining the correct Dilantin dosage. I shouldn't have anymore seizures which is definitely good. I will do anything not to experience another seizure. It was terrifying. I continue to feel stronger and am doing very well. Thank God!

March 21st: Wrote the following "Mom's Editorial" for the March Kelroy Gazette:

Life is a test. It is only a test. If this were your actual life you would have been given better instructions. Out of humor emerges truth. I want to thank all of you for supplying the answers which I found to be keeping the faith, never losing hope, and being open to love. Your prayers are heard, your hope gives us strength, and your love sustains us. The two individuals who have taught me the most during this time are Keith and Jason. If I can face life's challenges with the courage, faith, and humor Keith has shown and sacrifice for each other as Jason has for his brother I might not need better instructions.

March 21st: (Keith) It was a good day. Yesterday Dad and I set up my exercise bike. I rode it for five minutes. Man was I tired. I'm really concentrating on my hip. When I got off the bike, my legs felt so rubbery I couldn't believe it. I'm going to have a lot of work to do before I get back 100% of my functions. I will get back 100%. I'm confident of that. God gave me that confidence. Everything is going real well. Met with Dr. Cameron today, and we talked about my feelings at not being able to drive for three more months due to the seizure. I have not driven since Sept. 29th and that is hard, but by far not the hardest thing I've gone through. Losing cognitive ability has been the hardest. Took some cognitive tests today that I had taken back in November and found really confusing. In fact, I just couldn't do them back then. Today, they were just clicking, so it's coming back both mentally and physically. I've come to the conclusion as much as I want the physical back and I will get it back, my mental capabilities are the most important to recover. Going from the 99% on most tests to being average is hard for me to accept. Mom kids me that she's been average all her life and has found much happiness in life. She assures me life is very fulfilling without knowing how to do calculus. I told her the only way she could relate is to move her mental abilities to the low average range. I don't know how much longer I will be at Sacred Heart. Hopefully, I'll be back at Madison in a couple of months, or maybe a month the way things are going.

March 22nd: My husband's "Rite of Spring" was taking a bike ride to see all the new convertibles on the car lots. In the 26 years we had been married, every spring I have listened to him talk about owning a convertible someday. However, his someday always came after all of our todays such as paying for all the normal day to day money draining expenses of raising children, plus buying and maintaining a home, and paying for college educations which included my masters degree. Fred never put his desires ahead of his family and consequently had no "toys." At the time he was driving a four door used gray Camry with over 100,000 miles on it. Several years ago I began a super secret surprise savings account to give Fred a convertible the year of his fiftieth birthday. This was the year, and he was speechless when I told him his "Rite of Spring" was over. Now was the time for him to actually select a car and have it home by the Monday after Easter. Otherwise I told him I would pick one for him, which was a real scary thought because I know nothing about cars and could care less.

Fred and his sons took me seriously and really enjoyed spending their nights test driving and selecting the perfect car. Fred still says it was the happiest time in his life since all this began. Each night they would decide what dealership to visit and after test driving the vehicle spend the remainder of the night discussing the pros and cons of the car happily showing me the material they would bring home. I laughed when Keith told me a Corvette was not for Dad because Keith was embarrassed when they were passed on a two lane highway while test driving the car. The boys thought Fred was acting like an "old man" when he wanted to try out the new Chrysler convertible. However, after test driving it they changed their minds and were pleased when Fred settled on the new Sebring, which proved ideal as we could all comfortably ride in it. The first time I saw the car was when I went to write the check out for it so Fred could drive it home.

March 23rd: (Keith) I noticed my smile today. The right side is holding really well, and I can almost close my right eye and wink. I even had right sided facial movement like lifting up my cheek. In fact, I was working so hard at raising the right side of my face while it was drooping, now that it is not drooping at all I have a new problem. When I smile that side of my face is actually going up more than the other side. So now I have to look in the mirror to straighten out my smile, but that's just fine. I feel better now that my Dilantin level is squared away. I'm back down to three pills where I was before the seizure. My vision isn't blurry anymore. I was a little bit confused on the higher dose, and now I just feel a hundred times better. I'm anxious to see what my level will be this Wednesday. I'm guessing it will be between 10 and 14. Again, I'm doing really well, I'm just tired tonight.

March 24th: Our life had finally achieved some level of normalcy. Keith had improved to the point where Jason began to work part-time at the trust company where he had been employed last summer. They were wonderful about letting him determine his own hours, so he was always available to take Keith to his various appointments. Fred and I were at school on a regular basis. Fred's secretary kidded him now that he was showing up regularly she would need to put the visitor button she kept on his desk away. Keith was in the routine of going to therapies and continuing with his exercise program on his off days. He had also taken over all his own paperwork and was organizing his medical records, bills, and payments. I had been able to begin doing some volunteer work. In August, a family in our church had quadruplets, and there were numerous parishioners helping out with their care. I was enjoying the opportunity to help with supper and bedtime routine one night per week.

As Keith was improving Jason was becoming a little more assertive and some sibling conflicts were beginning to arise. One of the biggest sources of conflict was over the fact Keith had lost the concept of time which annoyed punctual Jason. He was never a patient waiter, but he did develop the coping strategy of giving Keith about 15 minutes lead time from the time he told Keith to be ready and the actual time he expected to leave. Still there were occasions when Keith felt Jason was rushing him which annoyed Keith and really irritated Jason.

March 24th: (Keith) Once again I'm much stronger. I was able to ride the stationary bike for 15 minutes really concentrating on my form. I feel steadier doing stairs and no longer need to use the railing going up or down. Cognitively things are much better, getting the Dilantin level straightened out was an improvement.

When I was over 20 I think I was having some toxicity. I did have a scare today. The left side of my lip started to tingle a little bit. All the negative memories started to come back with a vengeance. I had to tell myself anytime something goes wrong I'm going to have to fight the fear the disease is coming back. I was just so scared. I had to work at getting my mind off of it and when I did the tingling went away. I know the disease is not coming back, and I don't want to deal with fear for the rest of my life. I will have to really work at getting that under control, and I believe I will with time. I don't want to be playing basketball and have something happen to my right side and immediately panic that it is the disease returning. It will be hard, but I'm sure I will be able to conquer my fears. Right now this whole experience is still so fresh in my mind. I'm doing well though, real well.

March 26th: Except for Keith's seizure at the beginning of the month this had been his best month since September and therefore ours also. Spring had arrived and along with it came a rebirth of hope in my heart that everything would turn out fine. My friends at school decided our family needed to eat nutritiously and established a schedule to send me home with fully prepared meals. One was better than the next, and we were becoming spoiled. I started to regain some of the weight I had lost. One night I was the last one done eating when Fred asked about my weight. I told him I was gaining about a pound to a pound and a half a week. Without missing a beat he responded, "Oh, that's 52 to 75 pounds in a year." I chuckled and thought easy go, easy come.

April 2nd: (Keith) I've taken a little hiatus from talking into the tape recorder. I was at Phil's over the weekend, and I didn't bring my recorder down there. Overall I've continued to improve. I was able to jump for the first time and stand on my tip toes. I have more finger coordination, and I'm walking much better. My stamina is good. I'm starting to cook for myself and do my own laundry. Basically I'm self-sufficient. I'm even getting anxious to drive. Sat behind the steering wheel today and tried to work the brake and gas pedal. There is still pressure behind my right eye which is somewhat aggravating. Each day the mail still brings reminders people haven't forgotten about me. Of course it also brings my latest bills. The grand total is now approaching $100,000. Thank God for the wonderful insurance I have. I'm especially fortunate that I am not limited by a directory of doctors and hospitals. I believe I have been treated by the best of the best and have no desire to look any further for answers, but there is a sense of security in knowing that the decision to pursue further medical treatment is mine not my insurance company's. Looking forward to flying to Kansas City for Easter. Wrote an insert to put into our Easter cards.

I hesitate to write this letter because every time I have had good news it has been followed by bad news.........But this time is different! I have been improving for five weeks now. Previously the longest stretch of improvement was three weeks. I am now walking 3.5 miles and riding a stationary bike. My right arm and hand is constantly improving and my stanina is getting better daily.

I feel as though I finally beat this thing. But the recovery will never be fast enough. Whether it is two weeks or two years it will not be fast enough for me. So I just need to be patient. Ha!!!!! Those of you who know me understand that patience is not my strong suit, but determination is.

I want to thank everybody again for all their support, concern, and prayers. You cannot imagine how much it meant to me. There were many times throughout this ordeal that I felt like giving up. But every time that thought would creep into my mind I would think about everybody counting on me to get well.

Sincerely,

Keith Kelroy

Keith Kelroy

Easter 1996

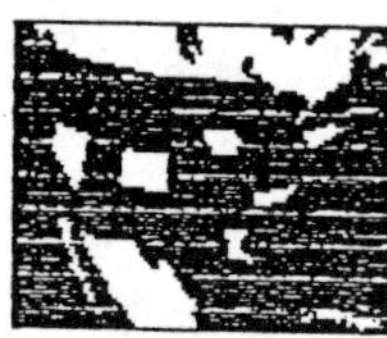

If memory serves us correctly our first newsletter went out around Halloween. At that time Keith had detoured from the road of rapid recovery. As you know since that time he has been mapping out a challenging route that has included numerous stumbling blocks, detours, and circular paths that have often led him back to the start of his journey. He asked for directions from numerous sources and eventually found himself in uncharted territory that took five weeks to cover. He's climbed the mountain, walked through the valley, and now is on level ground. So as we prepare to celebrate this Easter season we do so with grateful hearts. So far the journey has been long and often rugged, but we never felt abandoned for you traveled with us and because of Easter we knew we were never lost.
Fred and Karen

CHAPTER TWELVE

Mayo Clinic - Rochester, Minnesota

April 4th: Baptized Lutheran, confirmed Lutheran, married Catholic, recon-firmed Catholic, and rebaptized Baptist qualifies me for the label unorthodox Christian. If getting into heaven was dependent on documentation I was certifiable. My father's mother was a Quaker, and I believe Grandma passed on her faith to me. A faith that manifests itself without the constraints of individual sectarian doctrine but is based on an adherence to Biblical statements. As C.S. Lewis wrote in the preface to his book <u>Mere Christianity</u>:

> I offer no help to anyone who is hesitating between two Christian denomina-tions...I am a very ordinary layperson...the questions which divide Christians from one another often involve points of high Theology or even of ecclesiasti-cal history which ought never to be treated except by real experts. I should have been out of my depth in such waters: more in need of help myself than able to help others.

Even though I have always been comfortable with my personal faith, being part of an active faith community has always been extremely important to me. Therefore on that Holy Thursday I chose to be rebaptized to become an official member of Grace Baptist Church. It was not my "rebirth" because I have been blessed with the gift of faith for as long as I can remember. In my personal history there is no set moment that I can clearly identify as to when Jesus Christ became the pivotal force in my life. Believing has never been an issue, trusting has been. Holy Thursday, before a community of believers including Fred, Keith, and Jason, it felt appropri-ate to proclaim, even in tough times, my hope and strength comes from the Lord.

April 9th: (Keith) I've been lax as far as talking into the tape recorder. Probably close to a week since I've talked. When things are going good I tend to forget to tape. I talk into it when things are going bad because there is nothing much else to do. I continue to improve. I'm now using my right hand to eat, and I'm also start-ing to write with my right hand. I'm at my uncle's in Kansas City, and today I got lost walking in the neighborhood. I walked 2.6 miles in hilly terrain. I know because my cousin and I drove it afterwards to find out exactly how far I walked. Came home and even felt up to doing some push-ups. Down to 4mg of Prednisone. The vision has cleared. Things continue to go in the right direction. I'm looking forward to going to Mayo's next week to show them what I can do. I think they will be pleas-antly surprised if not ecstatic. That's about it for tonight. Okay!

April 10th: My mom was blessed with seven grandchildren, all boys, and her first great grandson had been born in February. We felt it was important that they meet so we offered to drive Mom to Kansas City over our spring break. Nathan

Russell Mitchell whose middle name was chosen in honor of my father, Russell Mitchell, was introduced to his great grandmother on this date. Keith had flown out earlier, and not surprisingly Jason had opted to spend the week in Madison. When Keith met us at the door looking tan and physically fit, I couldn't help but break into a smile. What a difference since we left him at that same door in late December. I agreed with Keith, his recovery since Christmas had been miraculous, and so had his attitude been throughout this whole experience. He continually energized us all with his fiery spirit. Even when he was alone with his thoughts he consistently recorded positive messages.

April 10th: (Keith) Talked to my boss yesterday about the letter I recently sent him. Once again it is a great company I work for because he told me there is going to be no pressure to come back to work. He certainly understands I need time to think. I may come back to Quantum or I may not. I just expressed I need time to think. When the doctors tell me I can go back in some capacity I will need to make a decision. As far as my boss is concerned, he just wants me to keep in contact weekly or at least every other week. If I decide not to return I will fly to Cincinnati to see the people in the corporate office and personally thank each of them. I haven't made up my mind yet. I work for a great company, and my boss has been extremely understanding. Just telling me I can come back, no strings attached, or I can quit, no strings attached, shows what a man of character he is. I really just don't know what I am going to do. I need to think what direction my life is going, what direction I want it to go. This has changed my life no doubt about it, and I'm not sure where it is going to lead me, but I'm sure God will take me in the right direction.

April 15th: After school I drove the two miles to Milwaukee's Mitchell Field to pick up Keith meeting him curbside after he had retrieved his own luggage and independently made his way outside the terminal. Three months ago, with the bitter cold north winds blowing, my brother flew home with him, now with the warm spring winds at his back Keith was finally flying solo on an apparent smooth course towards recovery. I remembered the verse from Ecclesiastic 3:1: "To every thing there is a season, and a time to every purpose under the heaven." I prayed this was finally now our time for healing.

April 16th: (Keith) In the car with Jason. We are returning from Mayo's after a one day follow-up appointment. The reports are very good. They are extremely pleased. The doctors said they could not have hoped for more. It has only been six weeks since the treatment, and I continue to improve. There has only been one other person who went through the study and improved this much totally, and I have done it in a month and a half. They are very pleased. Now they are putting me on a med-

ication to reduce my spasticity and stiffness. They think that is most of my problem right now. My strength is coming back so fast. It's not quite normal, but it is pretty near normal.

April 17th: (Keith) I saw Dr. Cameron today, he agreed things are definitely going well. I'm sure I'm going to get better. In fact, I'm sure I'm going to make a 100% recovery. Today I entered all my checks writing right handed, went through 30 or 40 pieces of mail, made phone calls to my insurance company and the Social Security Office. I took care of all of that. That may not seem like a big deal, but that is a long way from where I was six months ago. I could never have handled all that without being on overload. I would get confused. This weekend I'm heading up to Madison with Jason to check out the bars for the first time in over six months. Looking forward to it, but only N.A. beer. That's it!

April 20th: Jason and Keith were both up at Madison staying at Jay's apartment. Jason called from Carrie's to say Keith was tired and really didn't want to stay out late so he had returned to the apartment. Keith loved fun and in the past he was known to be the last one in on a Saturday night. Therefore, for Keith to want to call it an early night was unusual. Jason wondered if it was okay to leave him there alone. I told him yes realizing we would all need to learn to honor his desire to return to an independent lifestyle, but had to admit it was easier to relax when he was with us and we knew for certain he was okay. Knowing Keith was doing better did not mean he was fine, there were still obvious physical problems and subtle changes in his personality and mental functioning. For instance it took him longer to do everything, so taking care of his personal needs still consumed most of his time and energy. Yet he seemed eager to regain control of his life. I felt his desire for independence was encouraging because it was when things were going wrong he always wanted at least one of us by his side.

April 23rd: (Keith) I'm doing fantastic. Writing faster, walking three miles a day on a regular basis, foot is moving better, and my fine motor coordination continues to improve. Wednesday I dropped to one mg of Prednisone. This weekend Jay and I are going down to Beach Party at Champagne, Illinois. Hopefully it will be a good day, nice and sunny. I have been to five of them and it has always been great out. Short weather, always in the seventies or low eighties, so hopefully the trend will continue. I'm going to also stop in to see the head of the Campus Honor's Program Friday. I feel really good, I mean really good. That's the scoop!

April 29th: The guys arrived home from Beach Party partied out. They had stayed at Phil and Carissa's along with ten other guys. Jason said at night the living room floor was literally body to body. Today was Jason's 22nd birthday, and we celebrated with his favorite meal of pork chops with apple stuffing, which is always served with a retelling of the recipe's origin. A few years ago my brother and his family were coming for Christmas, and I wanted to create a memorable meal. I had decided on center cut pork chops. Prior to the holidays a store was having a special one day sale on them, but I was unable to shop due to school conferences. Fred volunteered to go for me which made me nervous as he is not good in the grocery store or the kitchen. After reviewing my limited options I hesitantly agreed. I kept stressing the fact I needed 18 perfect pork chops and he needed to ask the butcher to personally cut them for him, indicating they were to be served for a special occasion. All day I was apprehensive about the outcome of Fred's shopping expedition and thought about calling him to tell him not to bother, but I didn't. When I got home Fred told me he had good news and bad news. Immediately I knew it would be all bad news. He said the good news was he got the pork chops, but the bad news was by the time he got to the store the butcher was gone. However, he felt he was very lucky because there was only one remaining package which he purchased. My heart sank. The top five pork chops were picture perfect, but the next 13 were a mangy mess. One was so bad even Fred laughed when I held it up as it resembled an octopus with meat tentacles hanging out in all directions. No way could I use them for a special dinner, but the cost of the package forced creativity. First I cut them all up into boneless pieces. Then I located a pork and apple stuffing recipe which I substituted for my Christmas Eve dinner that did turn out to be delicious. Since then "Fred's Meal" has become a family favorite and is often requested on special occasions.

While eating dessert, following tradition, Jason shared the three best and worst things of the year. For him the best things that happened were being accepted into the law school at Madison, his vacation in Florida with Carrie, and making the Dean's List last semester. The three worst things were the day of Keith's surgery, the day he withdrew from law school, and the day of Keith's seizure. With Sam barking along we sang in our off tune manner Happy Birthday to Jason and wished him a better year.

Following dinner we talked with Keith about his future plans. I knew he wanted to believe he was going to continue to improve, but I was sensing a hesitancy about wanting to commit to plans for the fall. I was afraid Keith really didn't believe he would recover so it seemed important to continually let him know I thought he would. Therefore I encouraged him to take over Jason's lease. Jason's apartment was in a perfect location in regards to the business school. Plus it was on the first floor and really close to the gym where Keith would be able to go and work out. I was concerned that if Keith waited until August he would not be able to get a place close to campus that would meet his needs. As long as he had decided he wanted to return to school I thought he should translate his plans into action.

April 30th (Keith) Hello and once again I continue to improve dramatically. I now use my right hand to eat about 90% of the time. Once in awhile when I'm really feeding my face, I'll need to take a break and switch to my left hand, but that is happening less and less. I raced walked for the first time over the weekend. I was crossing Lincoln Avenue and almost got nailed by a car. That's one way to get me to run. Good to see everybody down there at Nabor House. I just felt normal this weekend. Cognitively and mentally I felt normal. I'm completely off Prednisone. I continue to take the medicine for spasticity, and it is working. I'm starting to notice a decrease in spasticity and tone. Within the next week I plan to go to a parking lot with Mom and Dad and see how the reflexes are and all that. I decided I'm going to school in September. Most likely part-time for the first semester. I just took over Jason's lease. His apartment is an efficiency and real close to the business school which we think would be better for me initially. Things are falling into place. I have received Social Security and Long Term Disability. So, hopefully, I'm not going to have to take out any loans. I'll graduate debt free with my savings I've accumulated, Social Security, and Long Term Disability. But you know what? I have been through hell and I've earned it. Social Security is not going to be there when I'm 65, so I might as well use it now. Yeah, I'm just feeling real good. Now I'm looking at my recovery as a challenge. Some people have doubts I'll ever play basketball or run again, not my family or friends because they know me. But some doctors do, and I am going to prove them wrong and I look forward to doing it. I realize now it is not going to be a fast recovery and it could take up to two years. But you know I keep my eye on the goal, and I know I can achieve it, as long as I don't get frustrated with the little steps. As long as I wake up tomorrow and do a little more than yesterday, I will be happy. I am just thrilled that I get a second chance at living with all my body parts working.

CHAPTER THIRTEEN

Sacred Heart - Milwaukee, Wisconsin

May 12th: (Keith) I had my team conference today at Sacred Heart. Those days are bum days. Every team conference I've had I've felt bummed after. Feel a little sorry for myself, a little depressed, but that will be all over tomorrow and then back to work. You know every time I have one of these team conferences I realize how much is left to do. I still can't run, I still can't play basketball. Then I listen to this tape and realize what I couldn't do two months ago, and then my spirits are lifted and I am ready to go. I have no doubt I am going to make a 100% recovery, but the task is daunting. I've got to see the big picture. I have to look two years down the road and see what I can do then. It's hard. I'm not a patient person, I never have been. I had an appointment today with Dr. Cameron, and he really feels this is not MS. I mean really feels it is not going to come back, it is a one time event. Now it's just a matter of how much I recover. I can look at everything I still can't do or look at the things I can do. Usually I look at the things I can do. It's just every now and then I get pissed off. Tonight is one of those nights, but I'll wake up a lot better tomorrow and then back to the grindstone. Rehab, rehab, rehab. That's the deal. Looks like I'll finish up before July. The people at Sacred Heart are really helping me. I'm improving every day. They tell me I'm improving very fast, but it doesn't seem fast to me. I need a lot of patience to get through this. Now the hard part has just begun.

May 13th: (Keith) Yesterday was a sucky day. About once or twice a month I start feeling really sorry for myself. Really down, but then right after the mood passes it's back to the grindstone. Yesterday was one of those days. I broke down in front of the psychiatrist. I just cried for awhile. I was all pissed off at life, at everything. It was good to get it out. The realization that I am far from normal is upsetting. I'm far from where I used to be. It is hard to admit that. Now I am average at everything I do. Not everything, I shouldn't say that. Things used to come so easily for me. It is a test of my true character to be able to deal with this and make the necessary changes and alterations to my life. I really do not believe there will be any permanent changes in my life, or if there are they will be very minimal ones. I hear about a friend I have made here at Sacred Heart who's projected recovery is ten years and I think how is he going to do that? I mean I'm pretty much normal now. I figure I only have to go two years for a 100% recovery including stamina. Today was a lot better. Friday was a bad day for a culmination of things. I have been having this headache right above my right eye. I think it is because I am awake more hours of the day, and I am putting strain on my right eye. It is not a bad headache, just really annoying and it wears on me. I put a patch over it today, and it was instantly better. I'm going to the eye doctor Thursday. I'm going to see my other doctors on Wednesday. I would like to think that eye glasses or contacts would take care of the

May 16th: Jason and Keith were really at each other. Jason was preparing to move out and return to Madison. He had reached his limit of togetherness and was anxious to leave Racine. He had secured a summer position at Four Lakes Driving School in Madison, but he needed to go through a 40 hour training program and pass an exam from the state before he could be certified as an instructor. He wanted to get that done before his summer law classes began and he was feeling crunched for time because we had asked him to stay and drive Keith to Sacred Heart that week as Fred and I were double booked with school commitments. Jason was not a happy camper, so I had requested Keith to please placate him.

After all Jay had done for us I wanted his departure to Madison to be positive, but Keith just could not resist insistently kidding him about any and everything. Keith's spontaneous kidding personality was wearing on Jason as he was not in the mood for his humor. Jason responded to Keith's wit with wisecracks which only escalated the situation. I had made numerous suggestions throughout the night including taking their disagreements outside to no avail. Finally, I lost my calm and emphatically told them to "STOP IT!" I told them they were both at fault, and I was equally mad at them. The dog does not tolerate any noise so he was irritatingly barking as I was lecturing. I scolded him too.

Then I went to simmer in a long hot bubble bath, mumbling as I went down the hall they were too old to act so young. After my bath I informed them I was going to bed and did not care to see or hear from them for the rest of the night. That did not make either one of them happy, and they camped outside the bedroom door lobbying to be able to tell their side of the story. Finally, I told them I would not listen to two sides of the story because I had heard more than enough bickering for one night. I suggested if they wanted to positively communicate with each other and come up with one story that had a happy ending I might reconsider letting them in the bedroom. Fortunately, in our family, anger does not sit comfortably among any of us, and we usually work towards fast and effective solutions during times of conflict. They were still upset with each other, but they were able to put that aside because they did not want me upset with them. Soon they were both in bed with me, along with the dog, and we all ended up laughing about their childish interactions and my overreaction.

May 19th: (Keith) Past week has been pretty amazing. I drove last week for the first time. Took Dad's new automatic convertible out to the church parking lot. Started there, then came back and went through the subdivision. As the week progressed I was driving on regular roads and the freeway. Yesterday I drove stick for the fist time. That went extremely well also. I just drove in the church parking lot, but I never killed it. I was in to see an optomologist because of the pressure and headaches. My vision is perfect. The problem is the muscles in the eye are trying to focus as well as the left eye so they are having to work harder. My headaches are getting better. I am not noticing it as much. It appears it just took time for my eyes to adjust to my increased awake time. No problem. Jason is out of here today. He is going back to Madison. He was a heck of a guy to come home and take the semester off. I just look back over the past eight months, and I don't know how we all got through it. I am very thankful for my family, Jason especially. He saved my parents tons of time from having to take off work to run me to therapy. He's great in a crisis. He stays calm, but when it is over he just wants to leave and that's that. But that is all right, he was there when I really needed him. I'm getting my life back in order. Now the hard thing will be making it through the summer and I don't think it will really be that hard. When you have a seizure you can't drive alone for three months. I can start driving alone June 11th. I'm planning on going to Kansas City for a couple of weeks. Then in July I'm basically gone for the whole month. I'll be in Wyoming and Colorado. When I come back it will be August and I leave the middle of August to reacclimate myself to Madison. I will go through orientation week and that sort of thing. It seems like such a long, but short, eight months. I wonder how I got through this. It was a combination of a lot of things. I had great family support.

People go through tragedies like this every day, and they don't always have the family that I had. The friends, prayers, my will, positive attitude, all that worked in my favor. I refused to give up. There were times when I was depressed from medication and /or the illness, especially about a month or six weeks after it happened. I was just really really depressed. I just didn't know if I would get my life back but then I'd focus on what happened during surgery. I'd remember that feeling. I can't explain it. It was just a warm feeling coming all over my body and an assurance that things were going to be fine. But it was such a long haul with all the ups and downs that I had my doubts, but not anymore. I'm going to be just fine.

May 23rd: Life was hectic. School was extremely busy with end of the year projects, reports, programs, and meetings. Keith had determined he would need a car and a computer for school, so our nights were busy helping him. Keith and Fred dealt with researching and leasing a car, but I was helping him select a computer. Keith wanted to go to Best Buy to look for a computer. The one we went to had a man picketing out front with a sign warning people not to buy from them. I pointed out the warning, but Keith said not to worry he was just looking. After becoming familiar with their stock we went to a local book store to do some comparison reading on the different brands and models. I convinced Keith to do some more looking, so over the next couple of nights we went to a few other stores which could not match the price and capabilities of the Acer he had found at Best Buy. That night he called his friend Phil out in Colorado to ask him his opinion. Phil told Keith he was really pleased with his Acer's performance, and Keith then decided that was the computer he wanted. I was okay with the computer, but uncomfortable buying it from a business with Lemon Man walking back and forth in front of the store. Fortunately, I wasn't the one writing out the check for it.

May 24th: (Keith) I figured out why I'm always pissed off on Fridays. That is when I meet with my psychiatrist. Right now he is testing me giving me certain concentration tests, and I'm scoring average on them. That pisses me off to no avail. I wasn't average before and I certainly don't want to be now. You know what is funny is my psychiatrist knows the kind of person I am, which is an extremely competitive person, and he is going to push me. He pinpointed me after three months as to the kind of person I am. Most people go through life being average, but I guess it's different for me because I was always way above average and now I'm average. That's like an average person finding themselves in the lower 5%. Usually it just takes an afternoon for me to stop feeling sorry for myself. Tomorrow I will be just fine. I'll wake up tomorrow, do exercises, math, writing all anew. You know I'm realizing that I am going to get better, but it is going to take every ounce of strength and determination that I have as a person. It would be so easy for someone to just give up and not keep up a good attitude. That would be the easiest to do, but it is not what I want to do. On a good note, played ping-pong today and my recreational therapist lost - he is a good man. Played for 45 minutes. Forehand and backhand both getting better. There is no doubt I will go to school in September, but I'm realizing that is going to take a lot of effort too. I may have to prepare myself in the back of my head to go part-time. I'm He Man, Superman - not true. I'm afraid I'll have to start with part time and gradually work into full time.

May 27th: We went to Best Buy to purchase the computer. When we drove in the parking lot the same man was still picketing out front. At that point Fred and I decided to purchase the extended warranty and give it to Keith for his upcoming birthday. As we drove out of the parking lot I wondered how many times we would be back. I just hoped I wouldn't have cause to want to join the man picketing.

May 27th: (Keith) What a day it was. I just shelled out $3800 dollars for a computer. That hurt. I almost made it four thousand. I got pulled over for speeding with my parents in the car. I was driving Dad's new convertible, and I was so flustered at having spent so much money I didn't hear the fuzz buster go off. I wasn't going any faster than traffic, but he must have caught me in a spot where I was accelerating. He said I was going 68 in a 55 mile per hour zone. When he pulled me over my mom was taking off the fuzz buster, and he said on his fog horn, or whatever the loud speaker is called, "Don't bother, I already saw it." Mom was flustered. He came up to the window and took my license. When he came back to the window he said, "Well Keith you were going 68 in a 55 mile hour zone, and that is a $118 ticket. Cars out here are going 65 which is way too fast. Sixty is one thing, 65 is still another, but when you approach 70 you are going to get a ticket." Then he told me to slow down, have a safe day, and walked away. I was so amazed I stuck my head out the window and said, "You mean you aren't going to give me a ticket?" He came back and said, "Why, do you want one?" He then gave me some fatherly advice about fuzz busters. He said when a cop pulls you over and sees one of those they are going to react in one of two ways. They are either going to laugh or get mad. He would recommend getting a CB which is what he uses. Then he told us to have a good day, and I was on my way. I am excited about using my computer. I have a month to learn it by typing some letters and doing stuff like that. Over and out.

May 29th: After dropping Keith off at Sacred Heart I headed back to Best Buy, once again encountering picket man. The night before Keith and I had spent several unsuccessful hours hooking up his "very easy plug and play system." That morning I had gotten up early to once again dial the ever busy 800 support number. When I actually reached a real person he walked me through numerous computer prompts reaching the same conclusion Keith and I did, the hard drive was defective. When I returned to the store the people were extremely nice about exchanging the computer which was good because I was not the cheerful customer. However, the technician told me he did not have time to reinstall the software to see if this computer would function properly as he was in the middle of a lengthy repair. I observed what he was doing which appeared to be just continually striking the F key along with the numeral 4 key. I asked how long the repair would take and he estimated an hour. I inquired if all that time would be spent pushing F4, and he said basically yes except when an occasional message would come up on the monitor. I told him he would look twice as efficient if he repaired two computers in an hour. I then offered to stand right there, free of charge, and faithfully and efficiently push F4 notifying him of any on screen changes if he'd reload my hard drive. He accepted my offer and now "Computer Technician" can be added to my resume. Within an hour the second of eventually three new hard drives was properly loaded and ready for Keith's use. I returned to Sacred Heart just as Keith was done with his therapies. With the writing of this book the computer and I have developed a meaningful relationship. Initially when I received the prompt "hit any key to continue," I thought of using a hammer, but we have resolved many of our conflicts and now interact pretty effectively.

May 29th: (Keith) Today was a down right shitty day. My mom was frustrated. I was frustrated at the way things have been going. I know I have been healing incredibly fast, but it just frustrates me that all this happened. None of this should have happened. Today I just felt like quitting, the hell with it. It's not worth it. I can't do it anymore. Tomorrow morning I'll get up and do it again. I'll go through my home program of rehab, use my computer, do some filing. I go on. I'm like the energizer rabbit and just keep on going, but I'm human and I'm going to have days like these. Fortunately they come about once a month where nothing seems to go right. I only have two more weeks before I can drive alone. Things will be much different then. I'm looking forward to it. I am going to get better and recover completely and totally. I just need to keep my eye on the target, the big picture. A year from now I plan to be completely, totally back. We'll see. I may be disappointed, but I need to set a goal. I'm going into it with the idea I will be back, I will never ever give up. I will keep my eye on the target I am trying to achieve which is total and complete recovery. I'm down to therapy just once a week. Originally, the improvement was so dramatic. It is still coming quite regularly, but it has slowed down. It is not as noticeable which in a way is good because the noticeable things came fast. Playing basketball is going to come slow. Running again, things like that, that is where my determination will count. I have all that, I just forget sometimes.

May 31st: It was my birthday, and following tradition I reflected on the three best things and worst things of the year. For best I came up with trusting my faith, Keith moving to Madison, and Jason making the Dean's List. For worst it was St. Mary's - Madison, St. Mary's - Rochester, and St. Mary's- Racine.

CHAPTER FOURTEEN

St. Mary's Hospital - Racine, Wisconsin

June 10th: (Keith) It is a big day. I started driving alone. Last week I leased an automatic Toyota Corolla. I can drive stick, but I wanted to be able to go and not have to worry about the clutch and shifting gears. This way there are only a gas pedal and a brake. I just got back from a weekend at my friend's in Ohio. Had a great time, but it was kind of hard though. My buddy had to carry my bag on and off the plane. Someone had to help cut my steak. I remembered everything we did together less than a year ago, and I started to feel real sorry for myself. I really have to watch that. I have to avoid that at all cost. Otherwise, things are going real well. I'm a little frustrated about my muscle tone, I'm thinking about taking a shot that might help it. I'm going to talk to my doctors sometime this week for more information concerning the shot. I dribbled a basketball 65 times with my right hand. I'm playing pool and things are just looking up everyday. I've got to keep my spirits up, and I will continue to try and do that which is about the best I can do. I have the gift to be able to see long term. I know long term I will look back on this as just one big bad dream, but this nightmare can't get over fast enough for me.

June 11th: I did not hear Keith come in, but I knew he was home when I got up and saw his bedroom door shut. Ninety days had passed since his seizure which meant the driving restriction was history. We had driven his new car over to his friend's house for him to drive home. I imagined the sense of freedom he felt. Officially it was the second day of my summer vacation, and I had volunteered to help out at Vacation Bible School. When I got home, Keith and I visited about his trip to Ohio. He said he had a good time, but it bothered him to have to accept some assistance. He said he could never go through this again and hoped he had the patience to wait out this apparent long recovery. After awhile Keith decided to go out and dribble his basketball, so I got ready to meet my girlfriend for lunch. When I drove away he was heading outside. He still couldn't shoot hoops but was getting closer and believed practicing dribbling under the hoop was great motivation.

I returned within 90 minutes and everything appeared perfectly normal. The basketball was out, radio was on, and our dog was meandering around the front yard. I assumed Keith had gone into the house for something because he was nowhere in sight. I walked in with my usual greeting but received no response. When I reached the kitchen, I caught a glimpse of Keith lying in the hallway. He was conscious, but uncommunicative due to seizure activity. Somehow I kept my calm dialing 911 and Fred at school. When the paramedics arrived Keith still had not improved, so they transported him to the hospital. A few neighbors had gathered by the time Keith was taken out of our house having first become aware something was wrong when the ambulance came into the subdivision. Our neighbors contacted the church and soon Pastor Rusty arrived along with Pastor Jerry, the senior pastor. In many ways our lives have paralleled Pastor Jerry and his wife Jane's. We are the same age, married the same length of time, and welcomed the same number, but not the same sex children, into the world at the same time. Jerry and Jane minister to Fred and me in a special way because of our commonality of experiences. From this time forward the entire pastoral team became involved in our lives, in a deep and personal way, and we were cared for by all of them. Two medications were tried and both were unsuccessful in stopping the seizure activity. The emergency room doctor was concerned by the length of the seizure, so we reluctantly authorized a cat-scan to make sure there were no new problems, as he thought perhaps Keith sustained additional head trauma in a fall when the seizure first began. We were extremely hesitant to give our permission for the test because Keith had specifically told us, after his last seizure, not to authorize any scans because nothing would be wrong and he did not want to be exposed to the additional radiation. Keith was right, the cat-scan was negative. At that point a neurologist was called to the emergency room. By now several stressful hours had passed. After examining Keith he ordered the medication Ativan and sent Keith to the Intensive Care Unit.

Before everyone left I called Jason from the hospital and felt sick as I listened to him vomit before he could communicate with me. Now I understood what Jason meant when he said Keith's initial seizure was the worst day of his life because of all I had been through with Keith this was the worst. I felt totally helpless watching him lay there unsuccessfully trying to communicate because his speech was garbled, yet knowing he was processing something horrible going on in his brain. Eight incredibly long hours from the onset, Keith came out of the seizure. Even in the Intensive Care Unit, Fred and I never left his bedside, so we had been up over 24 hours. Lack of sleep coupled with emotional exhaustion and fear of the unknown made us emotionally vulnerable. I felt like a fragile piece of glass teetering on a shelf. If the glass fell it would shatter into so many pieces there would never be any hope of putting it back together. I was still together, but getting closer to the edge.

June 13th: (Keith) It's been an interesting week. Where do I start? Tuesday I had a seizure, the first day I could start driving. I just can't believe it. I will go through the details. I came in Tuesday, June 11th, from dribbling a basketball. By the way, I dribbled 155 times. I came to the bathroom and my arm started to go crazy. About 30 seconds later, I realized I was having a seizure and lowered myself to the floor. I was conscious but unable to stop the seizure. At first I thought I was going to die, but then realized I wasn't and tried to relax. Mom came home about a half hour or 45 minutes later, and I was still in the seizure. I was rushed to the hospital in an ambulance and kept overnight. I was scared, mad and I don't remember too much about it because I was given a drug to relax me and a side effect is amnesia. Mom says it's good I don't remember much after getting to the hospital.

June 14th: That morning Keith found me sitting out on our deck enjoying a cup of herbal tea taking in the warmth of the early morning sun. I was desperately trying to get my act together. When I saw him, I wished him a Happy Birthday. He began crying as he told me he was afraid the disease was returning. My 24 year old son crying on his birthday was about as far from the good life as one could get. I contacted his MS specialist who agreed to see us. I then called Fred home from work as I just couldn't face the possibility of hearing any more bad news alone. The doctor was reassuring in the sense that he doubted a seizure could reactivate demyelination, but did believe due to the length of the seizure there could be some residual effects on the nervous system for a few days explaining the tingling Keith was experiencing. Before the sun set on his birthday we asked Keith the three best things of the year, and he told us moving to Madison, winning the 3-on-3 Hoop It Up Basketball Tournament, and backpacking in the Rockies. The three worst were the day of his surgery, the day of his first seizure, and the day of his second seizure.

June 14th: (Keith) My birthday! Today is my birthday and, just like Christmas, it sucks. I was supposed to go out with my friends, but they brought pizza over because I am still wiped out. Plus, I've started to have some tingling which is really freaking me out. I just have to keep hanging onto the idea I am going to be fine. I was told that. I can never deny that experience. Obviously I didn't know how long it would take. I still believe I will be fine. I swear to God I will be fine. I need to write the book.

June 16th: (Keith) Hello! I've had some tingling in my appendages. My doctor said that is normal after a seizure, and the demyelination is not coming back. Even after the seizure I have more strength than the last time I saw him. Even though I'm weaker from the seizure, my doctor still smiled at the improvement. He is not all that worried, and so I guess I shouldn't be either. What started off as tingling on both sides of my body has now changed to hot flashes. I'm trying not to worry, but I think about it. I also think about how I had this feeling during surgery that I was going to be okay, so I have to trust that. I have to realize no matter how long it takes I am going to be okay. I need to accept that it is in God's control. It is kind of a good feeling.

June 17th: (Keith) You know God has blessed me or cursed me, and I don't know which one, with an incredible desire to live. I am not afraid to die, I am just afraid to suffer. If I keep getting better then I can wait out this recovery, but I can't go through this again. I know I am going to go to heaven, so I am not afraid to die. I really believe in God so I am not afraid to die, not at all. Yet I feel like I have more to do here, more to give. These last nine and a half months have really changed my life. My life will never be the same. I think by now most people would just want to

*give up, but gosh I don't yet. I'm cursed or blessed that way. I really believe deep
down this will all be over someday, but I no longer know when. I am willing to let
it be in God's hands. I don't need to explain it! I just need to accept it.*

June 19th: Ever since June 11th my stress was reaching a new and dangerous
level. I was afraid Keith was not okay and was a seizure about to happen, a thought
which petrified me. Everytime I walked down the hall I visualized him lying there.
Fred was concerned about me and encouraged me to use the day to try and get my
emotions under control. When he left to take Keith to therapy, I called the doctor's
office and asked to speak to the nurse. I told them I was a mother going out of control and needed to know if they thought Keith would have another seizure and was
assured they did not. After her words of comfort, I went out to work in the front
flower garden. Sometime later I glanced at my watch and decided I needed to go in
and get ready as I was meeting the Baby Bunch. For whatever reason, after my bath,
I only wrapped myself in a towel and proceeded to spot clean the carpet. I was down
on my knees cleaning the carpet when my neighbor rang the doorbell. I invited
Jackie in and realized a couple of minutes into the visit I was only wearing a towel
so excused myself to put on a robe. On the way to the bedroom I noticed I never
drained the tub. When she left, I discovered my garden tools lying on the front porch
which I'd forgotten to put away. I looked over at the driveway and saw she was able
to drive only partway in because I moved the garbage cans half way up the driveway instead of returning them to the garage. I shared those events with the Baby
Bunch, and they unanimously agreed it might be time for me to speak to a counselor
as my bizarre behaviors were screaming stress overload. I never had time to make
an appointment.

June 20th: Keith was concerned when he woke up with an unusual metallic taste
in his mouth. He had done some reading on seizures and discovered some people
have an unusual taste sensation prior to a seizure. Late that afternoon he called his
doctor who felt Keith's taste was not indicative of a seizure because of the length of
time he had experienced it. Fred and I had play tickets that night. After talking to
the doctor Keith appeared relieved and said he wanted us all to keep our original
plans. He was going to Matt's house, and we drove him feeling terrible his new car
was parked in our driveway. I cried on the way to the theater. Before the final act
we were called to the lobby. Matt was on the phone with the news Keith felt he was
going to have a seizure.
We immediately left the performance and found Keith on the floor at his friend's
house. He had not had a seizure, but was sure he was close to having one. Fred
called the medical answering service, and we returned home to wait for the doctor's
call. As the minutes ticked away, Keith was more confident a seizure was imminent,

so we got in the car and I drove to St. Mary's. Sitting in the parking lot outside the emergency room I had the strong feeling this was not where we were to be, and asked Keith if he thought he could make it to St. Joseph's which was a 45 minute drive away. Keith thought he could. The reason I wanted to go there was that's where his MS specialist practiced, and I felt if we had any chance of getting a handle on what was happening Keith needed to be in the environment where the man ultimately responsible for designing his treatment plan could personally observe what was happening. I knew I wanted Keith admitted to the hospital, I just hoped the emergency room doctor would agree with me.

This was an interesting emergency room as it really was two in one. Upon arrival Keith, like every patient, was given a quick assessment. As soon as we indicated he felt a seizure was coming on we were whisked to the emergency room for high priority emergencies. I had taken along his medical records from when he was treated at St. Mary's in Racine. When I showed them that Ativan was the drug that was successful, the nurse literally ran down the hall to the pharmacy to obtain the medication. Within minutes of her return Keith began to have seizure activity. I had to leave the room, or they would have had two emergencies to deal with. Fred stayed with Keith. The drug was immediately injected and fortunately the seizure stopped. His doctor was then called, who I personally talked to, and the decision was made to admit Keith.

CHAPTER FIFTEEN

St. Joseph's Hospital - Milwaukee, Wisconsin

June 21st: I left Fred and Keith at the hospital around two in the morning when Keith had stabilized and was being transferred to a regular room. To exit I had to walk back through the same emergency entrance through which we had arrived and noticed a room full of people waiting for their turn to receive medical attention. I doubt if I will ever complain if I have to wait in an emergency room, because I will realize my condition might be uncomfortable, but fortunately it is not high priority. I would have given anything to have switched places with those people and been sitting there visiting with Keith, impatiently waiting to be called.

When I returned mid morning, Keith was undergoing a series of tests including an MRI. The results were encouraging in that overall the scan showed a reduction of lesion size by approximately one-third compared to the scan performed at the Mayo Clinic in March. His MS specialist decided to add Phenobarbital as a second seizure medication and keep him in the hospital for observation. He told Keith some people need a second medication to control seizures, and he expected Keith's symptoms to dissipate once both medications were at the therapeutic level. The problem was it takes time to reach that level and up until then there was still a potential for seizure activity. He explained it is important not to be too high as that also causes problems, and had targeted a specific range where he wanted to see Keith's levels at before releasing him.

June 23rd: When Keith was released from the hospital he was on Dilantin and Phenobarbital with an additional prescription for Ativan to take if needed for the taste aura. Within the first six hours at home he experienced the taste sensation and needed Ativan. Once that drug reached his bloodstream he became extremely lethargic. Just the mention of him having the metallic taste in his mouth made me nervous.

June 25th: (Keith) A lot has been going on this week. I have had a couple of seizures and I am here to tell you about it. The doctors think, I reiterate think, they know what is going on. There is scarring from the healing that is going on in my brain, and that scarring is causing my brain to trigger focal seizures. They believe they can control my problem with medication, but it is all experimentation. They think they will find a medicine or combination of drugs that will work. In the meantime, they have given me a prescription to use whenever I get this funny taste in my mouth which is an aura. This medication halts the seizure and my activity for about four hours as it puts me to sleep. Good things have come about this past week. The seizures weren't very good, but I had an MRI that showed the disease was stopped. Halted! Non- existent! It is getting smaller which is great news. I had an EEG which showed no seizure activity in my brain, so the doctors should be able to take care of the area where I am having the problem. I feel I am on the final stretch. If we get this problem cleared there will be no more problems. I've started to jog, pretty pathetic jog I admit. I also shot pool and played darts. If I don't have to take the Ativan I have the stamina to do push-ups and sit-ups. No doubt, after that long seizure I came back stronger. My tone is even better which is something the doctors can't explain. I prayed for that, doesn't matter if they can't explain it, it happened. I had an eight hour seizure on the 11th of June and another seizure at the hospital on June 20th. However, that wasn't a big seizure. I developed this taste which intensified over several hours, so I went to the hospital. An IV line was started just as I began to shake and get aphasia so immediately they injected a drug and the seizure stopped 30 seconds later. They kept me for a couple of more days and now I'm back home. The doctor guarantees me he can control this. It is not the type of seizure that can't be controlled. It's just a matter of experimenting with drugs and finding the right one. I will do anything to not experience another seizure.

June 28th: We went to Madison with Keith so he could meet with a person from the McBurney Disability Resource Center at the University of Wisconsin. Fred took Keith while I spent the time with my mom. Later Fred shared Keith found it to be an extremely long, stressful, and depressing day. Being on the campus observing countless active healthy young adults enjoying the sunshine and freedom of summer made Keith painfully aware of just how physically limited he had become. He also knew letters preceded his arrival which documented all of his deficits. I could only imagine his mental torment as he reflected on the realization that previous to that infamous September day letters addressed his intellectual talents, physical abilities, all-around good character, and academic successes. In addition to emotionally dealing with what he saw and heard Keith experienced an aura prior to his appointment so was on maximum medication which made it difficult for him to physically function during the formal assessment. Then on the way back to Milwaukee he needed to take a second Ativan to halt an increasing taste aura. At that point we were trapped in a car, miles from a hospital, and I felt a sense of desperation. It was then I realized I was succumbing to fear, a paralyzing fear that was infiltrating every area of my life.

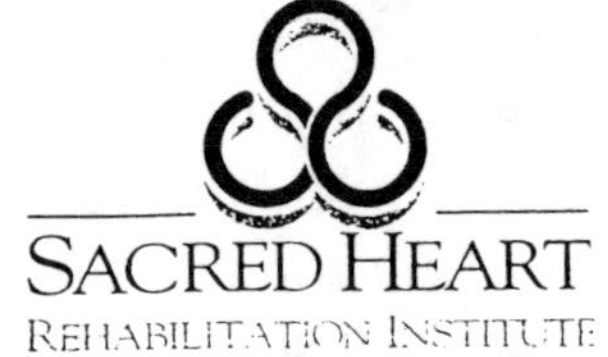

2350 NORTH LAKE DRIVE

MILWAUKEE, WISCONSIN 53211

PHONE (414) 298-6700

June 11, 1996

RE: KEITH KELROY

To Whom It May Concern:

Keith Kelroy is under my care as an outpatient for his condition of status post demyelinating encephalopathy. He has had excellent recovery from this condition to the point where he is now walking without any devices. He still has some weakness and spasticity of his right arm and leg, and he has not yet resumed driving. He has decreased strength and coordination of his right arm and he is right handed.

Mr. Kelroy developed this condition in the Fall of 1995. At his worst, he was unable to walk and had great difficulty speaking and finding words. The condition is now stable and improving. He has responded well to treatment and is no longer receiving treatment. The prognosis of this condition is for continued improvement.

Regarding how this condition affects student functions, Mr. Kelroy would have limited ability to carry things in his right arm, he does experience some difficulty concentrating and with reading, he has diminished strength and dexterity of his right upper extremity. With regard to exam taking, he may require extra time. He also may require extra time for walking long distances or climbing stairs. He also would have diminished ability to take notes because his right hand has been affected and he is right handed.

It is still uncertain whether his improvement will continue to the point that his disabilities become temporary disabilities, or whether he will have any long lasting or permanent disabilities from this episode of demyelinization. I am anticipating that he will experience at least some level of disability for approximately the next six months.

I last examined Mr. Kelroy on June 6, 1996.

Sincerely,

Jeffrey S. Cameron, M.D.

ln

Horizon Healthcare

Member of DAUGHTERS OF CHARITY NATIONAL HEALTH SYSTEM

June 30th: Keith and I were both having a really hard time. I dreaded being alone with him for fear he'd seizure. The taste sensation was increasing even though the doctor kept increasing the amount of Phenobarbital. When Fred, Keith, and I went out to eat Keith began crying. The year of the zebra he cried more than he had in his entire life. He said he had taken an additional Ativan because he was terrified by the thought of another seizure. He then sobbed out the words, "Why did you leave me that day?" It was a question I had asked myself countless times and always came up with the same answer. Because he seemed fine. He then fully described the experience of lying there helpless waiting for me to come home. He told us we would never be able to imagine how awful that experience was, and he would prefer death than having to live in fear of seizures. He spoke of his faith and belief that if his purpose on earth was to be a martyr then so be it. On his deathbed, he would still claim God told him he would be fine. He had no doubts his salvation was secure. Right now life was scaring him, not death.

July 1st: I had asked Fred not to leave me alone with Keith until the threat of seizures was past. That morning Keith and I were both downstairs. He was exercising, I was using his computer, and Fred was outside staining the cedar trim. The next thing I knew Keith was on his way upstairs and a few moments later I heard him slam and kick his door which to my knowledge was something he had never done before. I went upstairs and found him on his bed using uncharacteristically angry language which I also never heard him use before. He was livid over the fact the taste sensation had returned and forced him to take his emergency medication. Past practice had been within ten minutes of taking the medication the taste would fade along with his energy. He was filled with frustration at the thought of another four hours of feeling drugged.

However, this time after ten minutes instead of decreasing the taste increased, so I called Fred into the house as I dialed the MS specialist's office. I was told the doctor was unavailable. After waiting another 15 minutes Keith suggested we go to the hospital because he was beginning to experience the sensation of an impending seizure. We left immediately looking ugly with Fred's hair and skin speckled with stain, Keith in his never to be thrown away favorite ragged and torn U of I T-shirt, and me dressed in never to be seen in public clothes. The doctor's office was connected to the hospital and using the car phone we were able to communicate Keith's condition. The nurse had located the doctor who told us to come to his office. He was waiting for us when we arrived.

July 1st. (Keith) I'm back in the hospital and this time the doctors won't let me go home until the seizures are under control. I had the taste sensation this morning and even with a double dose of Ativan my symptoms continued to increase. I asked my parents to drive me to the hospital, but fortunately I never had a seizure. Now I'm hooked up to an IV line, so if need be, they can give me medication to stop the seizure immediately. The emergency pill I take has some nasty side-effects. It makes me tired, drowsy, and makes me feel drunk so I want off of it. I don't want to take the Ativan. Right now I am also on Dilantin and Phenobarbital. My current Phenobarbital level is 16.1. The therapeutic level is between 20 and 40, I need to get up to that level to see if it is working. If we get up there and I still have to take the Lorazapam, which is another name for Ativan, then we will have to try another drug. I feel we are on the right track. I don't believe I will be in this hospital again. I know we won't. Goodnight.

July 2nd: (Keith) I'm still in St. Joseph's for seizure prevention. I am here for observation. I keep getting a taste in my mouth which precedes a seizure. Until that taste leaves they are going to keep me. I heard good news today. Basically my MS doctor is done with me. I can just see him on a sporadic basis. Now it's up to me to see how much I recover. I am still getting better. Today Dad hooked up my basketball hoop to an IV pole, and I practiced shooting out in the hall. I'm doing well shooting with my right hand. It is unbelievable. The MRI shows the lesion has shrunk by a third since March. If the trend continues, it will be gone in six months. I am going to be transferred to Froedtert Hospital tomorrow to see a seizure specialist, but he already ordered a new medication which I've begun. Mom asked my doctor what side effects I might experience and he said the only one he knew of was possible stomach upset. I am now on three anti-seizure medications plus Ativan, so there is no way I am going to have a seizure. The doctors are going to have to reduce one of the medications, either Depakote, Phenobarbital, or Dilantin because together they make me real tired and with school we can't have that. I suspect they will reduce the Dilantin. At Froedtert I will be hooked up to an EEG thing that will continually monitor my brain waves to determine if the taste aura signals a change in brain waves. This hospital doesn't have that machine. I feel this is it. I feel this is the end. This is the last time I will be in the hospital. I really feel this is the end. I am going to make it through this. AMEN.

That was Keith's last entry and the only time he used the word AMEN.

CHAPTER SIXTEEN

Froedtert Hospital - Milwaukee, Wisconsin

July 3rd: Fred and I transferred Keith to Froedtert Hospital stopping en route to enjoy a picnic lunch. Surrounded by the warmth and colors of summer, we sat on the grass enjoying lunch and predicting how soon our lives would return to normal. Afterwards we reluctantly drove to Froedtert, and upon arrival Keith was assigned a single room. The environment was pleasant, as his fourth floor room was bright and sunny and there was a beautiful enclosed courtyard which provided ample opportunity to enjoy sunshine. Keith met with his new team of doctors and once again repeated his story. This hospital was different because it is affiliated with the medical college which meant whenever Keith was evaluated by his primary doctor several students would also be present in the room. The "teacher" would always arrive with numerous young people who would circle Keith's bed like Conestoga wagons around a campfire. We kidded Keith saying he needed an informational video like they show on airplanes prior to take off.

Keith was now under the care of a neurologist we knew nothing about except the important fact he was considered an expert on the prevention and treatment of seizures. He was an elderly man who appeared to take an interest in Keith, but did not seem overly concerned he was taking four medications for seizure control. I was. I had no idea how he could function on Dilantin, Phenobarbital, Ativan, and now Depakote. Keith told me it was because he was a machine, and he could adjust to anything. What we had to adjust to was the disappointing news the EEG machine Keith was sent to this hospital for was temporarily unavailable due to the holiday weekend and rotation change of the residents.

Jason arrived that night. While we were at Mayo's our family was invited to spend a week at a ranch in the Grand Tetons, and we had scheduled it for the week of July sixth. Fred, Keith, and Pastor Rusty felt it was important that Jason, Carrie, and I still make the trip. I was definitely the reluctant traveler. Fred wanted me to go because since Keith's last seizure my stress was increasing while my weight was decreasing, plus he knew how much Jason had looked forward to taking the trip, and felt it would be in everyone's best interest if we kept our plans. Carrie had been an incredible support to Jason during this whole ordeal, and he really wanted to show his appreciation by taking her to the Tetons. Pastor Rusty visited Keith that night, and later Keith called to say they both agreed the three of us were to go. Before we left, Jason wanted Fred and me to have a two day mini-honeymoon, and had purposely arrived early to stay with Keith. During the past weeks Jay felt Fred and I were not getting enough couple time so he would arrange dates for us, always making himself available to come and be Keith's support person. This time he really wanted us to have an overnight.

July 4th: Fred and I headed to Door County, Wisconsin and spent the day biking in Peninsula State Park. Fred was remaining optimistic that Keith's seizures could be controlled, and he'd be fine. I tried to relax and bask in the light of his confidence and sunshine of the day, but used the car phone several times to be continually told things were okay at the hospital. However, Keith was extremely tired. We called again that evening before we made the final decision to stay overnight. We visited with both guys who assured us everything was under control. Based on that conversation we located a place for the night, but our options were limited due to the holiday weekend. The resort we discovered had been open only three days, and all they had left was one suite with a spectacular view of Sturgeon Bay and an incredibly high nightly rate. At first, we declined to pay the cost of our entire original honeymoon on the one remaining suite, but then reconsidered our options, wrote out the check, called Jason with the phone number, ordered a pizza, and sat mesmerized by the spectacular sunset over the waters of Green Bay totally unaware of the shadow overtaking us.

July 5th: We awoke to the sound of the telephone. Jason had planned to spend the night at the hospital with Keith, but decided against it when his brother suggested he go home. The hospital discouraged overnight guests and Keith seemed okay alone. Jay was calling to tell us when he arrived back at the hospital numerous medical personnel were in Keith's room trying unsuccessfully to get him to respond. They were ordering an EEG. Jason said Keith was not only pretty unresponsive but also uncooperative, telling us he actually tried to hit him. We immediately left arriving at the hospital three hours later to find Keith's godfather and twin cousins there.

Jason was visibly upset, while Keith was basically uncommunicative, agitated, and disorientated. We were told he had an unwitnessed seizure and was experiencing the after effects. Having seen the aftermath of two previous seizures, I seriously doubted that diagnosis. Thus when his primary doctor arrived I questioned him about Keith's unresponsiveness. Obviously the doctor did not like my questions and wanted to prove nothing was seriously wrong with Keith so went over and twisted his ear in such an extreme manner Keith moaned in pain. I was livid and told him to stop. He then proceeded, in an pontificate manner, to inform me I was the one who wanted Keith to respond, and asked did I want any more response? There are no words to express my rage at that moment. I physically wanted to attack him. My brother-in-law, who witnessed the entire episode, said his veterinarian treats his farm animals better.

The day deteriorated from there, and I became emotionally distraught. A staff member present in the room at the time of the incident contacted a social worker who came to see me. She asked if I wanted to lodge a formal complaint, and I told her I needed time to sort it all out. What I really wanted was for Keith to wake up and be okay, and nobody seemed to be helping us make that happen. I certainly knew how Keith responded during the aftermath of a seizure having literally stood by him each and every time. I will always bear some guilt that I let Keith down that day, but the man rendered me powerless with his tongue and actions. What he did was not only unprofessional and inappropriate but began the cycle of events that took Keith's life. From that point on Keith was very restless but not alert. As day turned into night he seemed more comfortable and was starting to appear to settle into a relaxed sleep.

Around midnight Fred told me I needed to go home and pack for our trip. Jason was a wreck, feeling totally responsible for what happened because he chose not to spend the night at the hospital. The doctor who inflicted physical pain on Keith also inflicted emotional pain on Jason by telling him there was no way they could determine when Keith had the seizure because the hospital couldn't be responsible for people 24 hours a day. The doctor had the audacity to involve us saying we could not support Keith 24 hours a day which we were quick to retort yes we could and did depending on his medical needs. Fred or Jason had spent countless nights with him, both in and out of the hospital. After that brass comment, we made the promise never to leave Keith alone while he was at Froedtert. We requested a cot, and someone stayed with him from that point on. Fred said he could handle Keith, but he could not handle all three of us falling apart. Fred needed us to catch the plane. Jay and I arrived home after 1 a.m., and I reluctantly began packing.

July 6th: Fred called at five to say Keith was resting comfortably and we were to leave. Shortly after Carrie and her mom picked us up. I called Fred from the Milwaukee airport and he told me to go. I called from Chicago to be told things were okay, to eat, and have a good time, but as we were flying up and away, Fred's world began to collapse. The doctors determined Keith was not resting comfortably, but had slipped into a deep coma and was near death due to ammonia toxicity. The seizure specialist's willingness to attribute Keith's unresponsiveness to the aftereffects of an unwitnessed seizure instead of probing further into the cause sent him to the ICU with a level that was even medically unbelievable. At the time Keith was moved into the Intensive Care Unit, he had an ammonia level of 580 compared to the normal range of 40. With a level that high Keith had been suffering from ammonia toxicity on the fifth even as that arrogant and overconfident doctor assured us nothing was wrong. If the problem had been discovered when the level had been somewhere around 250 it would still have been serious but correctable, now Keith was at such a level the outcome was uncertain. When the hospital called in a metabolic specialist the first thing he did was have them repeat the test because he could not believe the level could reach that height, a fact he personally shared with Fred.

The remainder of the day was a living nightmare for Fred. Fortunately, there were "God sightings." My friend Lori arrived at the hospital and spent the entire day with him. Afterwards, she told me she had intended to visit on Sunday, but woke up early that Saturday morning feeling a sense of urgency to get to the hospital. As her husband and she already had plans for the day Dan suggested they wait until Sunday, but she was insistent about going immediately. Lori is the only other person we know of who experienced both the sense of peace and assurance Keith had that he would be fine. For her it occurred one spring night when she awoke thinking about Keith. She had gotten up and was sitting in a chair reading when the overwhelming sense of God's presence enveloped her. She told me it was so powerful it was unnerving in its intensity. Like Keith, after that night she was positive he was going to be fine. Lori would score well within the range of normal on any psychological evaluation, only what she experienced wouldn't. Therefore, when she sensed she was needed at the hospital she literally felt compelled to get there as fast as she could. She truly believes it was by God's intervention I was spared the pain of that day as she is positive I would not have survived as even calm Fred aged ten years.

Fred's sister Barb and his parents also came. Pastor Rusty arrived and brought along a doctor who specializes in internal medicine who helped Fred understand the information coming from all directions. Fred was well aware of Keith's advanced directives for end-of-life care, but felt there was hope Keith might pull through with aggressive treatment. Fred prayerfully authorized all recommended medical procedures while trying to reach us.

When we finally arrived in Wyoming, we were told Keith was in ICU before we were even out of the car. Jason's girlfriend has always been quiet and reserved in unfamiliar situations, and had only met our host at Jason's college graduation party, yet we immediately left her alone as we spent our time on four way telephone conference calls with Pastor Rusty and Fred. After the final phone call I went outside and gazed up at the mountains. Keith loved the mountains. Although he had skied and hiked many mountain ranges he had only been to the Tetons once before. In January, when Keith received the invitation he was excited. Making it back to the ranch was an important goal for him, and one he wanted to achieve.

Now I wondered if I would ever see Keith alive again. Were we trying to keep him alive and his spirit trapped in a body that was obviously failing him? I had more questions than the number of stars shining down on me that night, and most of them began with the word "what." "God, what is happening? What do you want us to do? What is your plan for Keith? What did you mean when you said he would be fine?" Some people had indicated they believed "The Evil One" was a force in this saga. I never resolved that issue. We certainly had experienced set back after set back, but sometimes I wondered if I was the reason because of my doubts.

I prayed, and certainly believed in prayer, but I never had the confidence Keith did that everything would be "fine." That day of his surgery I was never told Keith would be "fine." What I experienced was a peace that literally goes beyond description or my human understanding. A peace and an assurance that God knew what was happening in our lives. Years ago, a school psychologist nicknamed me Pollyanna as I always look at the bright side of life. In my bathroom I have a painting of a scruffy bear with her mop and scrub bucket looking into a mirror and what she sees is the reflection of a beautiful bear dressed all in white. I think, in some fuzzy way, I always felt what was happening here on earth reflected the scruffy bear and the bright picture was beyond.

From the beginning I held onto Keith like he had fallen off a cliff and was clinging to life by the rope I was holding. I held the rope as tight as I could, but try as he would he never was able to climb all the way back up. Just as he would get close, he'd slip back again. With each setback I was slowly losing my grip and some of my strength. Being at the mountains that night was a "God sighting." While Fred was in the hospital surrounded by medical help, I was remembering Psalm 121, and the verse about lifting my eyes to the mountain. Standing next to our host, gazing at snow capped peaks, I was listening to this man of wisdom suggest perhaps God was calling Keith home. I responded to his words by silently praying the serenity prayer, "God grant me the serenity to accept the things I cannot change, the courage to change the things I can, and the wisdom to know the difference." Later Jason made arrangements to drop off the rental car hundreds of miles from where we had expected to return it. Carrie and I laughed at how we had over-packed for an overnight vacation. I was glad she was with us.

July 7th: When we boarded the plane in Milwaukee on the sixth I told Jason that if he ever doubted my deep love for him, he would just need to remember this day because nothing, absolutely nothing else could take me away from Keith. I repeated the same sentiments when we changed planes in Chicago. The seventh confirmed my love for Keith as he was the only reason I agreed to board such a small plane for such a long flight. It was an eight passenger jet which our host graciously provided us a ride in as there were no commercial seats available. The jet was another "God sighting" as this was only the second time in over 20 years that our host had not flown commercial to reach the ranch. Fortunately, this "sighting" was extremely fast and within two and a half hours we had traveled the 1400 miles and landed safely in Milwaukee. Carrie's dad met us at the airport and drove us directly to the hospital. Upon arrival, we greeted most of Fred's family and thanked his dad for staying the day before and spending the night at the hospital with Fred. Then Fred took us into the ICU.

My immediate reaction was I was looking at the suffering Christ. On Keith's head were countless probes to monitor his brain waves which reminded me of Christ's crown of thorns. Because of a high fever, they had him on a cooling mattress, so he was striped of all clothes except for a small towel over his genitals. Every place Christ was punctured so was Keith with lines leading to various machines, plus he was on a respirator. I wanted to scream, "My God, my God, why have you forsaken me?" Instead my warm silent tears fell on him as I buried my head against his body in total and complete anguish.

Pastor Jerry and Jane arrived and I witnessed great sadness and sorrow in their eyes. Jerry offered a prayer, but no explanation for which I have always been grateful. I confirmed I knew Keith was a priceless gift from God. If for some unknown reason God wanted him back I would not understand, but I would try not to become bitter. However, if He allowed him to continue to suffer, I was afraid I might become an angry bitter person. Keith lived every day trusting in God's revelation, that he would be fine, and currently he was about as far from that assurance as he could get. I asked Pastor Jerry to please ask the church to pray for a complete recovery or eternal rest as it was time for Keith to be "fine."

The rest of that day was spent listening to doctors. For the first time I saw too many that wanted to talk to me and render their opinion. I asked each one about their faith and believed Keith was being treated by people of faith. I told them Keith was confident his salvation was secure and that would play a part in all decisions we made. Fortunately, the nurses accepted the fact we were a stay together kind of family and allowed us to move chairs into Keith's area where we kept vigil 24 hours a day.

July 8th: Dr. Cameron came to the hospital to see Keith. He did not have practicing rights, but came as a friend. He referred to Keith as possibly having a second zebra. That was the first time I ever heard the term "zebra" and asked him to explain what he meant. I told Dr. Cameron I was afraid Keith would be forever angry at us because everything being done to him was against what he had directed for end-of-life care. It was good to hear Dr. Cameron say he felt Fred had made the right decision by authorizing treatment. He believed Keith would pull out of the coma, and without any additional or new problems could recover. Keith continued to be unresponsive as we continually talked to him telling him we were waiting for him to wake-up. All doctor consultations were held at his bedside.

July 9th: For the second straight day, Keith had the hiccups caused by severe brain irritation. I hurt for him thinking what hiccup after hiccup must feel like. One doctor told us to try and imagine a gallon of ammonia sloshing in our brain, and we would have some understanding of the trauma going on in his brain. It was hard to comprehend as even the smell of ammonia is pungent and offensive to me. Keith began to show some voluntary leg movement, but otherwise remained unresponsive as we remained at his bedside.

July 10th: He was off the respirator partly because he removed it while they were taking an x-ray. They did not have to reinsert it because he was able to breathe independently with the support of oxygen. He was also more alert and tracking movements in his room, but he did not appear to be aware of his surroundings. He had begun saying "Oh my God" occasionally, but was not communicating with us. I could tell he was becoming medically stable because every few hours another tube was disconnected. At one point I had counted six IV bags delivering medicine into his body through various lines. Now he was down to just a couple. The doctors were encouraged by his progress, and we continued to hold all consultations by his bed.

July 11th: Keith was moved out of ICU as the Intensive Care Doctor wanted him exposed to less germs than were currently surrounding him. He returned to the same area where all his problems began and once again was under the original neurologist's care. Fred is extremely courteous and he had been able to maintain the lines of communication with that doctor. Fred felt he had no choice but to put his anger aside and work with the man as he needed his help in getting his son back. I had not talked to the neurologist except my first day back when he was part of a team meeting. My brother was with Keith when he was moved, and I was on the phone with Fred. I heard them go by as Keith was loudly repeating, "Oh my God." I told Fred those were my exact sentiments.

July 12th: Fred and Jason stayed at the hospital while I had gone home to try and sleep. After a very restless night I decided for Keith to get the best medical care intervention was required, so I wrote a letter. I never would have thought of writing the president of the hospital except his secretary had come to see me in the ICU to deliver a message that had come through his office. Within two hours of asking the social worker to deliver my letter the Chief of Neurology came to see us. First, he acknowledged mistakes had been made with Keith's case. He went so far as to say blood work had been done to test his ammonia level on July fifth. However, the laboratory disregarded the sample because it arrived improperly labeled. The test was never run until another blood draw was done on the sixth. What amazed me about that scenario was I was pressing for answers on the fifth. I kept telling the doctors something was wrong other than a post seizure reaction, yet no one thought to find out what happened to the results of the ammonia test. By the sixth, Keith's levels were so high he was close to death. The Chief Neurologist asked me what I wanted, and I told him, "My son back!" He told me that was the hospital's goal, and the seizure specialist identified in my letter asked to be removed from Keith's case. Fred and I were also told for the ammonia level to reach such a dangerous level there had to have been a previously unknown metabolic problem. While Keith was in the hospital we agreed to further detailed testing to determine the exact metabolic disorder he had. All the metabolic test results came back negative. Keith did not have a metabolic problem, the toxicity was apparently caused by the prescribed drugs that were not monitored properly.

July 13th: My brother spent the night with Keith and arrived at our home with good and bad news. The good news was Keith was showing signs of more voluntary movement, the bad news was during the night he had pulled out his feeding tube and took off his heart monitor. Phil and Carissa had moved to Colorado, and Keith had an airline ticket to visit them that weekend. Since Keith wouldn't be using it, the airline allowed us to exchange the ticket so Phil could fly to Milwaukee instead. We hoped seeing his fraternity brother would make Keith more alert and responsive. We also brought his framed picture collages from home to help him reconnect.

The doctors told us Keith awoke from the coma sooner than anticipated, but his mental capacities were not returning at the expected rate. All Keith kept saying over and over was, "Oh my God." It appeared he was having some form of hallucinations and was beginning to fight a significant battle between good and evil. Any spontaneous conversation had to do with religion. Late in the day Phil and his family were able to carry on a limited conversation recalling humorous happenings at Nabor House. Keith would follow their lead, but not initiate any dialogue. Fred's sisters Diane and Barb, along with Barb's husband Marv, spent the night with Keith. He was in a religious mode.

July 14th: My mother arrived unexpectedly and Keith looked at her in total fear. His reaction devastated my mom as they had always been extremely close. My mom was a source of comfort, wisdom, and love to him; pleasure not pain. For Christmas he had given her a pillow with the saying, "Thank Heaven for Grandma." It was difficult to determine who was more upset, and I did not know how to comfort either one. When she left I felt terrible, but decided I needed to stay and try to calm Keith down. It was becoming more and more obvious Keith was hallucinating. Later, Pastor Rusty visited and the nurses suggested he not talk about religion to Keith. I assured the medical staff that Keith woke up from the coma talking religion and it did not happen from any outside influence. Keith was in the middle of an internal struggle between good and evil which at times was manifested in him seeing the devil in people. Keith had been under the care of a wonderful aide since the day before he left the ICU, and I asked her to give me her honest opinion if she thought Keith was making any progress. She responded, "Oh my God." At that point you could hear our laugh down the hall because what she meant was most definitely, but her spontaneous choice of words were the ones she'd heard Keith repeat over and over countless times.

July 16th: Keith had stopped making progress, and in some ways had actually regressed. Even the aide who had told me she was seeing progress on the 14th said she was worried because he was not doing as well that day. The doctors said they were concerned.

July 17th: It was my turn to spend the night with Keith. Sometime after midnight he awoke very upset. A nurse determined his IV needed to be moved as irritation was present in its current location. I crawled in bed with Keith as once again pain was inflicted on him. Sometime later I fell asleep in his arms and awoke to his perfectly normal voice saying, "Hi, Mom." That was exciting. It was the same tone and inflection he always used when he was well. Then he went on to say in a very coherent manner, "God said you would protect me." I told him I would try and encouraged him to try and explain what he meant. As much I want to remember his exact words I can't, but the message was he needed to go to God to get well. It was like he had knowledge or an awareness of his condition that I didn't have, and he wanted me to understand what was going to happen. His medical chart was composed of countless pages documenting his condition, but he was giving me new information. I asked him if he was sure and he emphatically responded, "Yes." I shared that was between God and him, but promised our family would always be here for him. I told him he could go to sleep knowing he would either wake up in heaven or here with at least one of us by his side. He asked me if I would be okay if he left, and I told him I thought so. I assured him no matter what the future held I would always be thankful he was my son. He told me he loved me, and then slept for the next couple of hours cradled in my arms as I laid awake wondering and worrying about the meaning of his words and life.

July 18th: Because Keith was not successfully coming out of the coma at the expected rate another MRI was recommended. At first we were reluctant to put him through anymore testing because they would have to sedate him which was just what we felt he did not need. We wanted Keith to get the chemicals out of his system, so he would become more alert. I called Dr. Cameron to ask him his opinion. Initially he agreed with us, but wanted to talk to Keith's primary care doctor to find out why they thought an MRI was necessary at this point in his recovery. After talking with Keith's doctor and hearing his concerns Dr. Cameron thought the test was appropriate, so we agreed to it. In talking to Dr. Cameron we had decided if the MRI showed no change, we would transfer Keith to Sacred Heart Rehabilitation Hospital to begin rehabilitation as soon as possible. That afternoon when he went for the test I went home to change and try to get a couple hours of sleep. As I was leaving Carissa arrived. Phil had returned to Denver to work, but Carissa was still visiting family.

Fred called within an hour with the shocking news the MRI showed a large tumor near Keith's brain stem, and the doctors would like to meet with the family. I couldn't believe it, yet I could considering what Keith had told me, and the fact he was getting worse. I called Jason in Madison to ask if he wanted to be present as we faced yet another crisis. He chose to come, and we all met back at the hospital that evening. We requested the meeting be held in Keith's room hoping in some way he could be part of the decision making process. Fred was initially told the MRI revealed a tumor, but by the time Jason and I arrived for the conference another doctor disagreed and felt it was severe demyelination that had returned with such a vengeance it had progressed to the brain stem. Only another brain biopsy would confirm which diagnosis was correct. This doctor recommended another round of plasmapheresis. Keith just kept saying over and over, "God help me." We reviewed our options.

If we agreed to another brain biopsy, which was the surgery he had had in October, the results would only indicate a treatment plan. If it was a brain tumor, its proximity to the brain stem would eliminate surgery and radiation would be recommended to slow, not halt, the growth of the tumor. A brain tumor in that location would be fatal. Demyelination would confirm Keith did have Atypical Fulminating Multiple Sclerosis for which there was no cure. Either diagnosis meant his condition would only deteriorate. We were hearing his condition was worsening and was not reversible.

This was new information. We were no longer dealing with the acute crisis of ammonia toxicity we faced on July 5th. Plasamapheresis offered at best only temporary relief as both conditions were incurable. Keith's Advanced Directives for end-of-life care stated, "No heroics, don't continue treatment if full independent functional capacity is not expected to return and my organs can be donated." Currently, Keith's functional capacity was being strapped in a wheelchair that provided head support, walking with support on both sides, full care assistance in terms of bodily needs, and limited cognitive ability. Fred, Jason, and I had to face the distressing fact it might be time to act on Keith's directives in his Power of Attorney for Health Care based on what we were told, what he had written, and what he said to me the night before. In order for that to happen two doctors needed to sign Keith's directives.

We were now with the neurologist given this case after our disturbing conference with the Chief of Neurology. He really did not know Keith. I think he was frustrated with our interactions with many of the doctors, and empathized with us over the wrong and misguided information we had been exposed to since our arrival at Froedtert. I know he was angry with the doctor treating the toxicity who told Fred it was a tumor. However, when we asked that doctor why he thought it was a tumor, he replied, "Because that was the consensus of the people reading the MRI." Consequently, we never had concrete answers to help us. Now we were seriously discussing terminating treatment. It was a painful and emotional discussion for all of us, and Keith just kept saying, "God help me." What we knew for sure was Keith's condition had taken a drastic change for the worse. We decided all of us would seek whatever counsel we needed and would meet in the morning to finalize our decision. We left Keith's room with heavy hearts.

We asked Pastor Rusty to come to the hospital, which he did, and brought along another person who is not only our friend but an elder in the church, a doctor, and a parent who lost a son about Keith's age due to a car accident. We left Jason with Keith and went outside. In the courtyard the sun was shining. We stayed long after the stars came out. Sitting between physician and pastor we were facing the ultimate question of when do you stop treatment? Keith had identified a stopping point. The question facing us in our Garden of Gethsemane was, is this it? Based on what we all shared we prayerfully decided Keith could not get better, and in accordance with his Advanced Directives it was appropriate not to prolong the dying process.

While we met, Jason joined us with the news that Keith had an apparent period of lucidity. Jason asked him about plasmapheresis and he said, "No." He told Jason the same thing he had told me the night before: "No more." Carissa and Phil's mom were still at the hospital, so we asked Carissa to call Phil and ask him what he thought Keith would want us to do. Phil said Keith told him he could never go through this again, and Phil felt it was right to honor his Advanced Directives. It was a "God sighting" that He sent pastor, physician, son, and friend to help us that unforgettable night.

July 19th: We all met back in Keith's room. The primary doctor said he was comfortable following Keith's Advanced Directives. He said there was no need to involve anyone else. The decision was made. Keith would be moved upstairs the next day to St. Camillus, a sub-acute care floor of the hospital, and given a chance to declare himself. If he showed substantial improvement, plasmaphereisis was still an option without another brain biopsy.

That afternoon Dr. Cameron came over. After we visited awhile I asked Keith if he had anything he wanted to say to Dr. Cameron. He reached out his hand and said, "Thank you." There is no doubt in my mind he knew who Dr. Cameron was, and it was something he wanted to say to him. Dr. Cameron then asked Keith if he was sure he did not want to come over to Sacred Heart and try to get better? Keith responded, "Yes." Then Dr. Cameron asked him if he wanted to have plasmapheresis and Keith replied, "No." He then rephrased the same questions in a couple of other ways until it became clear to both of us Keith understood what Dr. Cameron was offering, and he was saying no more. Dr. Cameron walked me out in the hall and said emotionally he was having a hard time with Keith's decision, but intellectually he understood and did believe Keith knew what he was doing. Keith had played the game of life just as hard as he could, but apparently knew it was time to take his ball and go home. We both knew he was thanking his friend, and saying good-bye to his medical quarterback. Shortly after he left Penny and Vern arrived from Madison, and I told them we had activated Keith's Advanced Directives. I was afraid people would call us quitters. The last thing Keith would have wanted was to be called a quitter, but Keith somehow knew it was over. Once he told me he had to go to heaven to get well he never wavered in that decision and restated that fact over and over those last weeks. Penny and Vern comforted me with the thought it took unconditional love to love him enough to honor his wishes. Honoring his directives was unquestionably the most painful decision of my life, and if Keith had not so clearly told me, "God said you would protect me," I would not have made it through what was ahead.

CHAPTER SEVENTEEN

St. Camillus - Milwaukee, Wisconsin

July 21st: Keith was now in a nursing home, words that initially were difficult for me to say. I tended to just tell people he was moved to another room. In fact some people had trouble locating us, because when they would stop at Froedtert's information desk to find out Keith's room number they were told he was not there. St. Camillus had taken over a wing of the hospital because so many patients need additional rehabilitation, following a hospital stay, before returning to their own homes. The average stay is eleven days. Fortunately, for us, his new room was just one floor up from his room in the hospital, and the rooms were almost identical in size and design. I doubt if Keith had any awareness that a move ever took place as they moved him and his bed, and we decorated the room identical to his previous one. They also moved the cot for us.

Keith had now acquired a little more speech, and had reconfirmed he did not want any more treatment and he needed to go to heaven. On this day we had taken Keith to a large reception area because there were more than 20 people visiting that afternoon. Keith was very agitated, kept pointing at various individuals saying bye, and telling them in a loud authoritative voice to leave. It was uncomfortable because he was persistent, and would direct his piercing eye at whoever was seated on his left. Almost everyone tried to sit beside him, but he told them all to leave which they did, in tears. I was the exception as I sat next to him the entire time, but on the opposite side from where he was directing his attention. In fact from then on he would ask for me whenever I was not at the hospital which was amazing because usually Keith preferred any family member except me to go to the doctor with him. Somehow I must have successfully conveyed to him I was able to handle this, and now he always wanted me by his side. He was not the Keith we all knew and loved, or the Keith we knew that loved us. But he was still our son, brother, relative, or close friend and the love and pain felt in the room that afternoon was almost unbearable. I don't know if what he was doing was his way of saying good-bye, or if his brain chemicals were just so completely out of balance, but his behavior threw all of us off emotional balance.

Jason was scheduled to begin a five week law course and asked Dr. Blindauer if she thought he should withdraw from the course. She said it would be better if he did not take the course, so once again he withdrew from law school. This particular doctor was a resident and one of two residents that we requested stay with Keith when we changed his primary doctor. Dr. Blindauer had attended to Keith ever since he was admitted to Froedtert, and had been a part of everything that had transpired since his arrival. When she would speak she would look directly at you, and I came to read her piercing eyes as clearly as I heard her voice. She allowed herself plenty of think time before responding to questions. At first I thought she did not know the answers to my questions, but I soon realized the opposite was true. Her responses were both insightful and helpful. She was a listener and from my experience with countless doctors, the ones who listened to their patients were the best. While at Froedtert and St. Camillus she was the most professional, caring, competent, and empathetic doctor we dealt with. Dr. Blindauer truly viewed what was happening from Keith's perspective, and helped him in countless ways. She is wise beyond her young years.

That night I was staying with Keith when he woke me up in the middle of the night singing the ABC song in an extremely loud voice. He did the same song over and over for about 30 minutes, always rising to a crescendo when he reached the letter Q. I kept reminding him, to no avail, Q was for quiet. There was absolutely nothing I could say or do to convince him to stop. He was so noisy I was terrified we would be asked to leave, so I held a pillow slightly above his mouth to muffle the sound. Then I was afraid a nurse would walk in and think I was trying to suffocate him. At that point I just had to laugh at the absurdity of it all, and when he encouraged me to sing along I did. Eventually he just stopped on his own and went back to sleep.

July 22nd: It was a horrible, no good, very bad day and one that still conjures up disappointment, and disillusionment in one of Keith's doctors. A man whose interaction with me on this date will always, in my mind, be the personification of the Cowardly Lion in <u>The Wizard of OZ</u>. I believe him to be a good man and doctor, but one who lacked courage. The doctor I am speaking about is the neurologist who was now in charge of Keith's case.

On this Monday morning Keith had more language, but no significant increase in comprehension. For instance, when the group arrived for morning rounds, the doctor reminded him he had graduated from the University of Illinois and Keith said that was not true. He told him he had a biochemistry degree which Keith denied. Then Keith told them he did not have MS. I could tell the doctor was hopeful he would be able to engage in some meaningful conversation with Keith. When he asked him what he had, Keith replied, "masturbation." After rounds Dr. Blindauer returned and talked privately to Keith. As she spoke she looked at him with the same penetrating eyes with which she always looked at me. She asked Keith what he wanted, and he told her, "Unplug the machines." She told him he wasn't on any machines, and he said something to the effect you know what I mean. Keith then asked her what she would want if she was him, and she told him she did not know. I can still hear Keith saying, "Yes you do, unplug the machines." She continued, in a gentle manner, to probe Keith's mind and after a few more statements she came over by me and said she was comfortable that Keith wanted his Advanced Directives honored. She just needed to hear it herself, and said she would enter the conversation on his medical chart.

Sometime after rounds Keith's primary care doctor stopped me in the hall to tell me a team of psychiatrists would be coming to evaluate Keith and he had also contacted the ethics board. In total shock I asked him if we could go into a room so he could explain this sudden and unexpected turn of events. He stood there, in his blue scrubs, with coffee cup in hand, and told me he didn't have the time. He had time for a cup of coffee, but the hardest decision of my life warranted only a few passing remarks in the hall. At that point he totally devalued Keith and me. You talk about the weather in the hall, nothing of significance is discussed in public, that is taught in Education 101 and I would hope it is taught in medical school. It is paramount to positive patient physician relationships that doctors understand the importance of confidentiality. When he stopped me in a public hallway I was literally representing Keith because I was his Power of Attorney for Heath Care. I could not process what was happening as this was the same man who said on Friday he was comfortable invoking Keith's Advanced Directives and no one else needed to be consulted except those of us in the room. Now, in the corridor of the hospital, with people all around, I was told the rules had changed. I asked him why and he mumbled something about changing his mind.

I inquired if he had spoken to Dr. Blindauer who heard Keith say he did not want anymore treatments? I told him she had entered her conversation with Keith on his medical chart. He told me he had read it, and that might mean Keith was suicidal. The words Keith spoke to me came like thunder in my ears, "God said you would protect me." I cannot imagine anyone loving life more than Keith, or relentlessly trying to recover from set back after set back time and time again. I do not believe doctors should have the sole responsibility of deciding appropriate care or when to stop treatment. Out of anger I responded I would not allow them to see Keith. He told me to take it up with them and left.

Totally distraught, I called Fred and fortunately we had the presence of mind to make three important phone calls that day. The first was to our friend, the doctor, who was with us on the night we prayerfully decided to honor Keith's Advanced Directives. I wanted to know what would happen if we just said we were taking Keith home. He indicated that if we removed him from the hospital against medical advice and withheld treatment, we could technically be charged with second degree murder if Keith died. His advice was to meet with the ethics board as he was familiar with Keith's medical condition and anticipated the committee would support our decision to honor his Advanced Directives. Next I called my brother. He told me that in a business environment, the couple of times he found himself in a position where he did not know the playing rules and everyone else did, he lost. He recommended we become educated on the function and rights of the ethics board before we met with them. Thus, my third call was to a lawyer. He explained the role of the board and exactly what the board could and could not do. He also clarified for us that we were meeting with them as Keith's personal medical representatives. Therefore, the only issue was whether or not to honor Keith's Power of Attorney for Health Care.

He stressed the importance of keeping the focus on Keith's directives. The advice we received from all three sources was beneficial and intellectually prepared us for the events of the next day. It was impossible to become emotionally prepared.

July 23rd: Again Jason drove in from Madison to meet with the ethics board as he had been part of the decision making on July 18th and 19th. I was surprised by the sheer volume of people involved. There was a psychiatric team of about six or seven members whose purpose was to determine if Keith was indeed incapable of making his own medical decisions. The actual ethics committee consisted of five or six members. We found the day and process painfully long. First, they met with Keith's primary care doctor. I do not know if that included residents involved in the case or not. Since September our goal was to have Keith make his own decisions, so we requested the meeting be held in his room as we had on all previous occasions. I did not always agree with the decisions Keith made during the year, but I was always thankful I was the support person and not the decision maker. It was unimaginable that our family was in this position, and from my perspective the psychiatric team was evaluating the wrong person as I was the one losing my mind.

My first shock came when the people on the ethics board told us only the medical staff could bring concerns to the committee. What about patients rights? What about what happened to Keith on July fifth? I thought, was the ethics committee ethical? It was not right what happened to Keith, and he had no voice in the decisions made on the 5th. Now a doctor was trying to render him voiceless once again. I really don't remember much of the discussion we had in Keith's room, except when they said what made this so difficult was Keith's age. If he were older there would be no question. Talk about a double standard. Why would anyone want to sentence a young person to a prolonged death, but not an older person? When there is no hope of recovery age does not matter. I was relieved when they left. Jason returned to his summer job in Madison. Shortly after, several of Keith's fraternity brothers arrived and we took Keith out to the courtyard. Several hours later, while still outside, the psychiatrists came to tell us the ethics committee supported their recommendation that we remain Keith's medical representatives with his Power of Attorney for Heath Care. His Advanced Directives would be honored. I cradled Keith in my arms as Keith's fraternity brothers put their arms around me. I had protected my son!

July 24th: The events of the past week caught up with and overwhelmed Fred. He was a mental mess, thus I suggested he put the top down on his car and drive far, far away. I knew I would be okay because my brother was with me. My brother had been with me through numerous interactions with doctors, but he observed something that morning I will never forget. The neurologist who took us to the ethics board arrived with his usual entourage of people. Now he suggested we might want to transfer Keith to Sacred Heart. I knew Keith did not qualify for Sacred Heart because he was not going to receive anymore treatments. My son needed to stay right where he was. I told the doctor I could not discuss that possibility because I had just arrived at the hospital. I informed him my brother had spent the night with Keith, and I had not had time to be updated on Keith's current condition. After he left the room my brother said, "He's afraid of you." I have no idea if that was true, but my brother's words gave me confidence to act as Keith's advocate from that point on. After that morning Dr. Blindauer became primarily responsible for Keith's care. The neurologist never officially removed himself, but I think he decided to physically remove himself as much as he could from the case, which was the right decision for all of us.

Fred had driven to Fond du Lac to see his brother Tom. Less than a week had passed since a tornado ripped through the area. When his brother's family came up from the basement and looked out their kitchen window, their neighbor's house was in their farm field. Their own home sustained significant damage. A pole barn was destroyed, one third of their herd of cattle had to be destroyed due to injuries, and the damage ran into tens of thousands of dollars. On the ground below the barn was a recliner that had hit the upper part of the barn with such force it left the impression of the chair in the wood. While Fred was there, television camera men arrived to interview his brother for the Milwaukee evening news. Later, as Fred and his brother were driving around surveying the damage, Tom shared what they were seeing was not on the same scale as what his Godson and our family were experiencing. Hearing that made Fred more cognizant of the chaos the winds of change were blowing into our lives. We were being whirled, hurled, tossed and thrown by events that were out of our control, yet seemingly under our control. What Fred came to accept that day, long before I did, was we were not the destructive force, but minor players. We did not create this drama. Rather we were cast into our roles and were only reading the script Keith had given us.

July 25th: Medically, Keith no longer qualified to even remain in a sub-acute care area as he physically and mentally could not participate in the required therapies. I communicated with his insurance company, through his case manager, to determine our options. She was professional, knowledgeable, caring, and empathetic. Keith's medical bills had now exceeded $150,000, and all expenses had been expediently paid. Surprisingly, even with incredible insurance, our personal costs which primarily included phone, food, travel, lodging, and moving expenses, plus out of pocket medical bills were over $15,000. It became obvious to us how catastrophic illnesses without adequate insurance and savings could bankrupt a family. I was told Keith had a hospice provision which would pay for 50 days in a hospice. A possible solution, I presented, was for St. Camillus to declare Keith's bed a hospice bed and his insurance company to agree to that arrangement so we would not have to move him again. For that to happen the nursing home and insurance company would have to agree. As Keith said frequently, "Let's pray about it."

July 26th: A doctor came to see me. He told me he could not speak for the hospital, but wished he could. He believed the hospital owed us an apology for putting us through what they did. He said the staff agreed Keith would not be himself, nor recover, and we were doing the best thing. This doctor shared he could not imagine how we were able to hold up and had great respect for us.

Psychiatrists became important in Keith's care. They determined that Keith's brain was overproducing a chemical called dopamine which was causing Keith to experience a "split" or loss of contact with reality. They began the drug Haldol to try to control his symptoms which included hallucinations and delusions, blunted emotions, and extreme behavioral changes. You could actually see it in his eyes when his mood would change. In his lucid state there were still remnants of his personality. In his altered state he would become violent to the point he was difficult to control. On this day he told us he had become decapitated in a combine. He often thought he was in hell and wanted to get to heaven. The saying hell on earth took on new meaning.

July 27th: Keith was experiencing symptoms indicative of ongoing brain misfunction such as dilated eyes, hiccups, and small seizure activity, but Fred and I continued to allow anyone who wanted to see him to come and visit. Amazingly, friends arrived from all over the world. Fred had called both Morgana and Joe and Nuria. Morgana was in the process of getting a visa so she could come. Keith's middle school friend, Joe, had been studying in Germany and was ending up the summer traveling. When he received word of Keith's condition he immediately left Italy to come home. George, another middle school friend, was now working in Japan and when he heard he came. Mary, his high school science partner, returned from her medical studies at Tulane to spend time with Keith. Phil took off time from his new job in Colorado to visit, and numerous fraternity brothers from the Nabor House were regulars. His friends in the area like Matt, Andy, and Allison came almost daily.

We gave all of them access to medical reports as they tried to come to grips with what was happening. Many of their visits were marked with the realization Keith had lost touch with reality, but sometimes he would surprise us with his coherent statements. Occasionally, Keith would begin confessing the sins of youth. His friends would remind him that if he wanted to confess his sins that was okay, but please don't start on theirs. Phil had spent the better part of four days with Keith yet really experienced no meaningful interactions. However, one hour before he had to leave, Keith became very lucid, and we all enjoyed an hour of laughter as he entertained us with college stories. At the end, he turned to his friend, told him he loved him, thanked him for his friendship, and said it wouldn't be as hard on him as he thought it would be. When we hugged at the elevator, Phil told me we had made the right decision. He also said he was glad he came back and would always remember the last hour.

July 28th: It would be impossible to record all of Keith's interactions, but Fred did keep detailed notes for the doctors to help them determine the correct dosage of his medications. Keith's medical needs were changing so quickly his medicines were being altered daily. Here is what Keith said and did between 5:45 a.m. and 6:45 a.m. I realize it will be hard to follow, but it accurately reflects how difficult our interactions were with Keith:

"I can read that - Keith we are thinking of you." (Lights were out and that was not what was on the banner in his room.) Then he said, "Dad, I can read this. You are in our hearts and prayers."(That was correct) "That's a calendar. I can read it." Identified Dream Catcher and explained it. Shook his head on and off, wouldn't tell me what he was doing then continued talking, stopped and shook some more. Could squeeze my hand a little with his right hand but couldn't release. Said he was happy because I believed in Christ. He said, "Let me take some more medicine, some whipped cream, it'll make me better." Then he recited the insert in his Bible, and said he needed more whipped cream. I cuddled in bed with him, then he yelled, "You are Satan," and pointed to his leg. "One more day- this will be the 10th day-you can't hurt me anymore." Asked me to crawl back in bed with him. Nurse brought fresh water. He didn't ask for any. After she left, he said, "You believe in Christ. Is it safe to talk? I could use some water." (Drank) "How about another glass - no I won't have another. I'll talk to you in heaven. I'm leaving" (I asked him where he was going.) He replied, "To heaven." (I asked him do you want to go to heaven or stay on earth?) "Go to heaven. One more day. Can I talk freely? On Thursday" (I asked do you know what is wrong?) "People who believe in evolution will go to hell. Turn off the plug. Want to go to heaven to get rid of MS because I didn't get my directive done in time. Death directive-a directive of what I want done in an emergency" Upset he didn't get the book done. Doesn't want to stay on earth with MS. Wants Mom to write the book because he has faith in Christ. (I asked where are you going?) "To heaven, Mom will write the book using the typewriter. Dad you could never learn to use it."

Within a couple of hours Fred left, and his sister Diane, Keith's godmother came. We took over for the day, and spent the time trying to meet Keith's needs. When he began ripping off his Depends we allowed him to. I made the decision they would never be put on him again and they weren't. Keith had become fascinated with crosses. His friends, Joe and George, had given him the wooden crosses they were wearing when they came to visit. Keith always wore them, and I always wore a cross that I received as a gift during this ordeal. Once I put it on I never took it off, it is my badge of courage and code of conduct. That morning Keith wanted to touch my cross and when I leaned forward he grabbed it with such force he broke the chain and hurt my neck. That was not the first time he unintentionally used force on me. Earlier in the week he had grabbed my arm and squeezed it so hard he bruised it. Both experiences were painful emotionally and physically because I knew the real Keith would never intentionally hurt me. After Diane fixed my chain, which I still wear with the damaged hook, we went outside. When Keith said he wanted out of the chair we supported him as he walked around the courtyard, which was against medical advice. We stayed calm when he got physically sick to his stomach and also when he experienced lapses of consciousness. We interacted with him constantly at whatever level he wanted. Keith continued to revert to childhood activities such as singing the ABC song and playing the game, My Father Owns. When he was lucid he primarily talked about the importance of faith, and confessing one's sins.

At the end of the day Diane shared it was a good day, but there was no doubt in her mind we had made the right decision. Our families knew and loved Keith since his birth. All are faith filled individuals witnessing through their daily actions that their priorities in life are faith and family. There is a significant difference in the environments where we formally worship, but a commonality in our belief that Jesus Christ is the head of our respective households. Hearing our families tell us we were validating Keith's life and faith by honoring his directives meant more than the official piece of paper we received from the ethics board. All we knew for sure was Keith's salvation was secure, and if we erred in judgment we erred in Keith's favor because he was going to a far better place than he currently was in. The losers would be us. Any loving parent wants what is best for their child, so we were reluctantly, painfully and tearfully relinquishing custody of our son to his Heavenly Father in accordance with Keith's wishes. I did so with anger and faith as no parent should be placed in this position. I wanted to lay down my life for Keith, instead I was being asked to lay down my peace of mind by honoring his faith and life through validating his directives. Using Keith's own words I prayed "God help me," and then added "God help us all."

July 29th: The "Baby Bunch" is the type of support group every person should have the privilege of experiencing. Judy began a schedule so someone was always with me during the day. Sue and Barb would come on their lunch breaks joining us in the courtyard. Karen, Judy, and Jan were regulars. Jan's husband Wally always came along with her, and Keith would always ask them to pray with him, which they faithfully did. Keith also enjoyed having the <u>Bible</u> read to him, and people would take turns. Often Keith would say, "Read faster, faster." Each and everyone was a "God sighting."

Every morning, after Keith was washed and dressed, we would take him outside for several hours. Often others would join us, old friends from outside the hospital and new friends from inside. Keith enjoyed being out and hated when we had to return for his medicine. One time when just Fred and Keith were in the courtyard, Keith became so distraught and agitated when it was time to come in that Fred needed the assistance of several staff members.

July 30th: Morgana was still having trouble obtaining the visa she needed to come from Brazil. The hospital worked with us to obtain the necessary paperwork which was an example of the countless ways the people at Froedtert and St. Camillus supported us as we tried to support Keith. Keith was no longer receiving physical therapy, but the physical therapist came at least once a day to spend time with us and offer any assistance he could. Nurses and aides from the neurological floor would spend their breaks with us, going so far as to give us their home phone numbers. Residents gave us their numbers and would stop in throughout the day to check on all of us. The nursing staff was caring and attentive, accommodating us in every way possible. The hospital's pastoral staff and social workers were wonderful, and people in administrative positions understanding and helpful.

There was one aide who knew what a struggle I was going through and shared with me that her family made the same decision many years ago concerning her sister who died at the age of 18. She did not need to share the pain of that experience, but I will never forget her kindness in telling me we were doing the right thing. Another day a social worker found me in bed questioning Keith if he was positive he needed to go to heaven and get well. She told me he was, and what I needed to do was to let him go, and tell him it was okay. Her words gave me the strength to tell him with confidence and conviction what he needed to hear from me. A nurse shared a near-death experience and how angry she was over the fact she wasn't allowed to die. She told me helping Keith restored her faith because now she felt she knew one of the reasons she was brought back which was to help Keith get ready for the wonderful life ahead of him. Story after story, kindness after kindness, sustained our family.

July 31st: A palliative doctor became involved in Keith's care. Fortunately Dr. Blindauer was given permission to work with this man, so she could still be Keith's primary doctor. This gentle man was a doctor who helps terminally ill patients. We found him to be extremely kind and caring. He was gentle with all of us. Keith's insurance company was still working with Saint Camillus to have his bed designated a hospice bed so we would not have to move him to another facility. When we inquired about the possibility of bringing him home, his doctors said we would be overwhelmed as his medical needs were changing so rapidly. The thought of acclimating to another facility scared me, and I continued to pray we would not have to move.

The pastors from our church were phenomenal in the number of visits they made. It was a 56 mile round trip from the church, and they were there several times a week. At one point Pastor Jerry and I went to a room, and he just assured me the church does not believe in prolonging the dying process. I recorded those words in my mind and occasionally still play them. Even though I knew we were doing what Keith wanted it was still incredibly hard and painful. One night a nurse was talking to Jason about the amount of medication Keith was now receiving. They thought Keith was asleep, but soon found out he wasn't for when the nurse told Jason, Keith was at the level where they have people when they are on a respirator Keith became alert and emphatically said, "No respirator." At some level, even with all the dysfunction going on in his brain, Keith still knew he was choosing no more treatment.

August lst: Keith was having difficulty determining between the real and surreal. Often he would have us touch his nose to prove we were real. On this particular day he asked me if I was real. I told him I was. He then shocked me when he said, "If you are real moon me." I told him that was about the only thing I would not do for him. At which point he said, "My brother would do it." I assured him that I was not his brother and a kiss would have to do. He smiled and accepted the only alternative I offered. Each day Keith was so different and continually managed by an increase in medication. I kept asking the same psychiatrist over and over if he was sure Keith's behavior was not being driven by an overdose of medication. Patiently, consistently, routinely, and empathetically he would explain that Keith's brain was malfunctioning at such a rapid rate medication was the only thing allowing him any sense of reality. Once more, I revisited the idea that perhaps medication was the main problem. Without putting me down he indicated, in his opinion, that Keith was demonstrating a need for another increase, but what he would do was write the orders and have the increase available when I decided it would be best to give it to Keith. If indeed medicine was the problem, Keith would stabilize or improve throughout the day, but if that was not the case I could request the additional dosage at anytime. Within six hours I asked the nurse to administer the additional medication which resulted in Keith becoming more comfortable. Finally I processed the information he had shared with me several times. The doctor never lorded the failed results of my mini-experiment over me, instead affirmed me saying my questioning was a normal reaction given the circumstances. I inquired as to why I needed to question the same thing over and over and was told people process information when they are emotionally ready to handle it. I now accepted the fact that Keith's brain was self-destructing before my eyes. Increased medication was now our ally instead of our enemy.

August 2nd: There is a saying all dressed up and nowhere to go. I felt all angered up and had nowhere to go with it. Pastor Warren, another associate pastor from Grace, was a regular visitor, but we rarely got to visit as Keith had the uncanny ability to go into medical crises in conjunction with his arrival. Time and time again Pastor Warren would arrive as we were engulfed with doctors, decisions, and dilemmas, and he'd graciously retreat from the scene. The night before he had left a message on our answering machine asking for a state of the family report. I called and left a message saying I was really angry and didn't know what to do about it. I told him I did not even know where to focus my anger. Pastor Warren arrived at the hospital early that morning, and found Keith and me out in the courtyard enjoying the warmth of a perfect summer morning. Keith was temporarily medically stable and fairly lucid. Keith shared he was angry because he wanted to get to heaven. I thought good, at least one of us knows where to focus our anger. He wanted to know why he was still here, and Pastor Warren suggested because he might still need to minister to people here. That message Keith took a little too literally because in the end it was hard for Keith to let go because there were still unsaved people. It was their first long visit in awhile and they both enjoyed it.

We then left Keith with a friend and went to another table to discuss my anger. He surprised me by sharing the pastoral staff had been waiting for the word anger to surface. He assured me we all had a right to feel angry over the situation and gave me the focus I needed. He was right most of my anger was not at God or people, it was at the situation we were in. Being a caregiver is exhausting, and the hardest work I have ever done. I was on stress overload, running low on emotional, spiritual, and physical energy, and felt that I was about to crash and burn. My emotions were raw, and my body was screaming "Red Alert," but now that I had a focus for my anger, I was able to begin to defuse it. I connected the ideas, situational anger and feelings are neither right or wrong they just are, into a healthy monologue beginning with a litany of "It's Not Fair." I was steamed about the whole situation. Pastor Warren helped me release my pent up anger until it was back in the safe zone. We then went over to Keith and he said good-bye to Keith for the final time. Keith and I still had the same burdens, they just didn't seem as heavy.

When I got home there was a message on our answering machine saying Morgana had obtained a visa and had gone directly from the embassy to the airport. She was on her way and would be arriving in the morning. I went to Chicago to pick her up at O'Hare Airport. Seeing her walk up the ramp was like a breath of fresh air coming into an extremely stagnant room. All my married life I was the minority surrounded by males, even our dog is a male. The year Morgana lived with us I learned the special joys of having a daughter, and I could not have loved her more if she was my biological child. Fred said my voice resonated with a joy he had not heard for a very long time when I called to tell him the time of her arrival. On the ride back to Milwaukee we visited nonstop and soon were in the courtyard of Froedtert. Keith recognized her, but did not interact with her. When we went to the cafeteria Morgana emotionally began to unravel saying as much as I tried to prepare her, she was unprepared for what she saw. Mother-to-daughter we dealt with the flood of emotions built up in both of us.

August 3rd: Ginny and John came up to help. John and Fred had spent the night with Keith, and Ginny and I took over in the morning. Shortly after we got Keith outside he experienced one of his longest periods of lucidity which was extremely emotional. I kidded him about catching me unprepared. Ginny went to get us some Kleenex and returned with an entire roll of toilet paper. She felt what was happening was the pits and toilet paper was more appropriate. Keith talked about the book. I indicated I would take notes and he needed to express what he wanted included in addition to his tapes. He had three specific messages: First, he wanted everyone to realize Jesus Christ is real. He reported heaven is easy access, all you need to do is confess your sins and have faith. Keith assured us his faith was real and soon he'd be on his way and seemed completely at peace with that thought. Next, he wanted to tell young people not to engage in premarital sex. Being with him on recent occasions when he felt compelled to confess his sins I was sure this was the voice of experience speaking. Finally he wanted people to realize souls have no color, and it is important not to let outward color affect attitudes or behaviors towards others. He did experience loss of consciousness for short periods, yet when alert he'd check to make sure I had taken notes and would restate the same thoughts he wanted published. During our time outside we also had the opportunity to remember special memories created by him over the years. He referred to having a charmed life.

The previous night when our husbands were at the hospital Ginny questioned the idea of us being at the hospital 24 hours a day. She could not imagine how we could do it, or would be able to continue to do it. However, that afternoon when Keith said he was tired and wanted to rest and would either wake up in heaven or with one of us there, she understood. The knowledge of knowing he would never be alone was comforting and calming. I believe that is the real value of being able to be in your own home under such circumstances. Since Keith's ongoing medical needs removed that option we needed to create a home away from home by continually surrounding him with the love of family and friends.

Keith then gave us the wonderful gift of sleeping peacefully for three hours, a length of time that by then was rarely achieved, allowing us time to share as only the closest of friends can. Because so many people traveled this journey with us, we had the freedom to not only express our pain, but also the humor we tried to find along the way. For instance, friends chuckled when we inquired into who wasn't praying hard enough when we were hit with set-backs. Often they would even suggest names of people present which would begin a delightful and humorous dialogue. They laughed when we wanted to know who filled our name in the box for volunteers, without reading the fine print which said volunteers will suffer extreme anguish. They appreciated the humor when we shared our sticker shock at the cost of a funeral and offered humorous ideas for cost effective measures.

Keith's nap also gave us time to redefine our friendship in the knowledge that our lives were being forever altered. Fred and I felt it was important to tell people we still wanted to be involved in their lives and hear about their ongoing joys and tribulations of being a parent. We realized we had a choice to make. We could either grieve the future we would not have with Keith or celebrate the past we did have and derive strength from the wisdom of his own words that we would be together again. We elected to celebrate, and set our course in that direction. I shared Keith's funeral would be a service of celebration. There would be no visitation as people were invited to visit Keith now. Instead we planned a Remembrance Reception after the service with a private burial the next morning. We selected to have Keith's physical body buried next to his grandmother on a hill that overlooks the Kelroy Farm.

Keith woke up. Keith was the first person to tell me he needed to go to heaven to get well, so it was comfortable interacting with him on that subject. He never mentioned his funeral, so I never brought it up. For him, death meant a passage between worlds, and he knew he was either going to be with us, or in heaven. I doubt if he ever thought about his own funeral. Shortly after he awoke, Morgana and Jason arrived to spend the night and we left to join our husbands for dinner. As I walked out the door, I glanced back and smiled remembering all the great times my sons and daughter had together. It was a "God sighting" when she originally came into our lives and another one now that she was back.

August 4th: It was Sunday and it did not make a difference as we realized regardless of the day of the week a doctor was available who was familiar with Keith. Fred asked Dr. Blindauer if she ever took time off and was overwhelmed and humbled by the response, doctors were voluntarily choosing to keep someone on that knew Keith. By this time his medical needs were changing at about six hour intervals, so having access to staff was indeed another "God sighting." A doctor shared what was happening in this room was affecting people throughout the hospital, and we had the prayers, empathy, and support of countless people. The sterility of the environment was giving way to compassion and understanding. We were no longer as angry at those who we felt erred in judgment. We were being healed by the incredible kindness surrounding us. Without remuneration, the staff was treating our whole family in countless supportive ways. Keith's bed had been designated a hospice bed, but his room had become a center of activity. At night two people were now staying so besides a cot we also had an air mattress Jason had smuggled in, that the night nurses willingly maneuvered around in the cluttered room. Visiting hours were determined by our needs instead of a sign on the door. The only rule seemed to be, does it meet our needs?

August 6th: The palliative care doctor met with Keith's primary doctors, the nursing staff, and us to discuss the fact Haldol was no longer keeping Keith mentally comfortable. The recommended additional medication meant Keith could not go outside as it would be administered by continuous infusion delivered by a pump through a very thin needle placed just under his skin. Another side effect might be Keith would sleep continuously until his death. Realizing he was not mentally comfortable, we thought he'd prefer sleep. We had shared all there was to share, he could literally rest in peace. Before the drug was administered the chaplain met independently with the nursing staff and us. The needle was inserted by his stomach, and I do not believe Keith realized it was there because he never complained or tried to remove it. Shortly after the medicine was begun Keith's face relaxed and he enjoyed a very restful sleep. From that point on the medicine needed to be continually adjusted to maintain a restful state, but he never went into a continual sleeping pattern. We visited with him up until hours before his death.

August 8th: Because none of my clothes were fitting, I went to the store to buy a pair of shorts and slacks. I had been a size ten for years, and now size four was loose on me. What scared me was when I looked in the mirror I thought I looked fat. The word anorexic came to mind, and I decided I needed to force myself to eat. The only way I ever had an understanding of how thin I was is when I would hold up my shorts and visually see how small the waist was. However, I never saw myself the way clothes indicated or people told me I looked. My weight never went lower, but only through effort on my part, for at that point it would have been extremely easy to intentionally or unintentionally allow myself to physically disappear.

August 9th: Plans were being made in preparation for Keith's physical death. We wanted an autopsy performed in hopes of discovering some answers for ourselves along with the hope perhaps some new knowledge could be gleaned that might help others facing a similar situation. I felt bad none of Keith's organs could be used as prior to last September he was the picture of health, and I knew he would have liked to have given others a chance for a better life. The fact they did not know the source of his illness prevented the use of any of his organs, which spoke volumes to the seriousness and hopelessness of his condition. We authorized a living blood draw because they said that would provide more information. A social worker talked to us about funeral arrangements. She became emotional and said this was so hard for her because she had a son Keith's age and had told him about Keith. Her son said given the same scenario, he would expect her to make the same decisions. She wasn't sure she would have the strength, but knew she would have to find it after watching us.

August 10th: Jason and I went for a walk. Fred and I had shared what each of us would need once Keith died, and we wanted to discern Jason's needs. Up to this point fight or flee had been our choices, and I believe all of us fought valiantly. However, I knew once Keith died I would need physical, emotional, and mental space from people, places, and decisions and there was a significant chance I would select to go away by myself for awhile. Fred said he would need to reconnect and reestablish some routine and normalcy both in his personal and professional life. He wanted to go and do. With such opposite yet important needs we realized we would each need to map out our own route through the inevitable path of grief which was still ahead of us. We promised not to program the recovery route for each other and respect the choices we independently made for ourselves. We agreed to keep counseling as an option and said we would give serious consideration to it if either of us suggested it.

When I discussed with Jason his needs he indicated he thought he'd be okay, but could not be Keith and Jason. He needed to just be Jason. I respected his honesty. I have seen in school where the death of a child negatively affected the surviving siblings' relationship with their parents. What I have observed is either the children feel they must fill the space created by the death, or the parents become so consumed by their loss they become blind to the love of the children still around them. Jason was laying important groundwork. The worst scenario would be if Keith's physical death put our relationship with Jason in any type of emotional jeopardy. He had been there, for all three of us, from the beginning, and now we needed to be there for him and value and treasure who he is: Jason John Kelroy.

August 11th: Keith said he could not go to heaven because he had not saved everyone and the book was not written. I promised to write the book and reminded him Jesus returned to heaven before he had saved everyone, but named disciples. I suggested he might want to designate some people to carry on his work. He thought that was a good idea, told me to get a piece of paper, and then went on to identify 26 people he thought would make good apostles. Interestingly, out of the hundreds of people he knew, the majority were people I'd recommend for such a short list. Although I have the list I have shown it to no one except Fred and Jason. Those of you who would like to think you were named by Keith should believe you are and live accordingly. One of my favorite sayings is: The Only <u>Bible</u> Some People May Ever Read Is My Life. That gets me up in the morning, and pretty much sets the direction of my day.

Later that day the chaplain visited and recited scripture. The verse Fred and I were helping Keith say came from II Timothy 4:7, "I have fought the good fight, I have finished the race, I have kept the faith." We told him God was waiting for him to come, and now it was time for him to go. That afternoon, following a nap, Keith told me he was dying and wanted me to write down what he wanted done with his money. First he talked about Jason, then designated money to religious organizations and friends who would benefit from his generosity. What stunned me was we had not discussed money with him, and he came within a few hundred dollars of allocating what he had in his sizable savings account without ever asking me what his total was. He asked me to read him the list of apostles. At that point he removed one name and replaced it with another. The next morning he added a final name, which verified he gave thought to those he selected.

August 12th: Jason had spent the night, and in the morning when Morgana and I arrived we found the guys in intense conversation. Keith had not slept well and was telling Jason if he went to sleep it would be over, and it was hard to say good-bye. In his own words, "It took a leap of faith." The kindly doctor arrived, said he understood, and Keith was right, the end was near. Final good-byes were very difficult, and the doctor said he would talk to someone about how to help Keith. Jason and Keith said good-bye to each other, and Jason returned to Madison not expecting to see his brother again, knowing there was nothing more to say or do. In one respect, by withdrawing from law school, he had laid down his life for his brother and believed Keith would have done the same for him. They had defined brotherhood.

During the next two hours I realized part of Keith's emotional upheaval was brought on by the fact he was no longer receiving Haldol since for the past two days he could no longer swallow pills and no IV lines were started per his wishes. The dopamine level was obviously rising because for the first time in a week he saw the "devil" when a psychiatrist came to see him. It was recommended Keith receive a long acting shot of Haldol to keep the evil thoughts away. I agreed, but no shot was ever needed.

Keith told me he would miss me and wanted to know if I could go with him. I honestly told him I wish I could, but this was a solo flight. However, I would try to follow his example so I could join him in heaven. I took comfort in the fact he told me not to worry I'd meet him there. We talked about who he would meet. He named many people from biblical times to the present. I added Eleanor Roosevelt, and he said, "Mom, you've always admired her, and I'll tell her." She once wrote:

You gain strength, courage, and confidence by every experience in which you really stop to look fear in the face. You are able to say to yourself, I lived through this horror. I can take the next thing that comes along. You must do the thing you think you cannot do.

That afternoon Keith's continuous infusion was changed with the addition of a second drug. Soon after he began to relax and parents of a childhood friend arrived. Keith was to be their son's best man which speaks to the depth of their friendship. Shortly after they came, Keith asked Morgana and me to leave. I was surprised as he always wanted one family member with him. I asked if he was sure and he said, "Yes" so we went and had a Coke.

When we returned Keith was sleeping. I inquired as to what he said, and they shared he just wanted to go to sleep. Keith never awoke again. In retrospect I am quite sure he couldn't leave us, so we had to leave him. From the time he went to sleep until his last breathe was about 10 hours. One hour before his death Morgana asked me if I could take her home. She had been at the hospital 13 hours, was emotionally exhausted, and I don't believe wanted to be there at the actual time of his death. Fred offered to take her, but I asked him to stay. I drove her home, and when I arrived back at the hospital Fred was sitting on the floor as I stepped off the elevator. I said, "It's over," and he said, "It's over. Keith has gone home." We went to his room, and he still felt warm.

At first I was devastated to think I wasn't there and Fred was alone, but then I realized that is what Keith would have wanted. The majority of the 102 nights in the hospital were spent with just his father. Countless nights at home the "two buds" slept together. I am sure to the very end Keith drew strength and peace from the steady hand of his father on his shoulder and his quiet reassuring voice telling him thanks for the miracle of his life, and saying it was time for him to go experience the new life waiting for him. I visualized his earthly father's hand on his left shoulder allowing him to go and his heavenly Father's hand on his right shoulder inviting him to come. I can think of no better passage between worlds. After saying a prayer of thanksgiving for his life, we left his room and never saw his physical body again. To us it was a shell that housed his immortal and invisible spirit that was now set free.

August 15th: How should we remember Keith? How should we feel about the fact he is gone? What can we learn from his extraordinary life? These are the answers **Pastor Rusty** gave us at Keith's service of celebration of his faith and life.

We should remember Keith the way he was. He was the kind of son every parent dreams of and could be described as a smile from God himself upon our lives ... He was the kind of brother every man dreams of and few have the priv-

ilege of knowing ... Keith was so many wonderful things. He was the friend who always had a way of lifting us up. He was the relative who represented what family is all about. He was the fellow student who enjoyed life and enjoyed friendship. He was the coworker who always did his part and inspired the rest to do the same ... For me he was a brother in Christ who deeply desired to know God and explore His vast character ... He was a wonderfully complex and vibrant person who exhibited a zest for life even until the end ... Remember him for the blessing he was to all of us.

How should we feel about the fact he is gone. We should feel privileged to have known him. We should feel grieved that he is no longer with us. And we should feel joyful, knowing that Keith is experiencing gain as he looks into the eyes of His creator and is enjoying the fullness of heaven ... And there is tremendous comfort for us today in knowing that Keith is experiencing that joy abundantly right now. For Keith the struggle is over, and the victory is won.

What can we learn from Keith's life? Well there are many things Keith's life taught all of us ... But there is one shining lesson that I know for a fact Keith would like us all to remember. One of his favorite phrases during his last days was "May I speak freely?" Well, just a few days before his final coma, Keith told me that he really wanted to come before the church and do just that, speak freely, about his new relationship with God. In a way I think he is getting his wish today and I believe that if we could send a television camera to heaven right now and talk to Keith directly he would tell us all that the life we are all living on this earth is not all there is ... Keith knew Jesus Christ as his Savior and had trusted in His death on a cross to get him to heaven ... I know from Keith's own mouth, that he knew he would be in heaven after he died, and because he knew that fact, he was not afraid, in the deepest parts of his soul, of death ... As Paul states in 2 Timothy 4:7, so Keith can say now: "I have fought the good fight, I have finished the race, I have kept the faith." May we all be able to say the same thing at the end of our lives.

AUGUST 16TH (FRED): THERE IT WAS ON A 4x6 CARD, BLACK ON WHITE, TWO LINES WRITTEN IN KEITH'S OWN HANDWRITING. I WAS AWAKENED BY A PRESENCE OF A MESSAGE FROM KEITH THE SATURDAY AFTER HE PASSED AWAY. OH, I DON'T GET A LOT OF "GOD SIGHTINGS" AS WE CALLED THEM DURING KEITH'S ILLNESS AND I DON'T DREAM OFTEN AND NEVER CAN REMEMBER ANY OF MY DREAMS. HOWEVER, ON THIS PARTICULAR MORNING I FELT THE PRESENCE OF A MESSAGE FROM KEITH. I STRUGGLED TO HOLD THIS VISION. NOT WANTING TO LOSE ITS PRESENCE, I TRIED TO SAVOR IT AND TRIED TO CAPTURE IT PERMANENTLY IN MY MIND. ON THE CARD WERE WRITTEN THE WORDS:

"Thank you Dad, for helping me out. I am fine."

Honoring Keith's Advanced Directives meant we would have him with us for a relatively short period of time. A miracle would have been nice, but Keith's recovery was not meant to be. Instead, as it turned out, Keith was the miracle. Some felt we should have ignored his directions and held out for all the "miracles of medicine." I felt Keith wanted quality not quantity. From time to time Keith had shared with us that he felt he could beat this thing once but didn't ever want to experience it again. During his coma I painfully gave permission for kidney dialysis. It was painful because I felt Keith didn't want any heroics done or any machines attached. Yet, the doctors felt there was a good chance that dialysis could pull Keith out of the coma and even bring him back to as good, or better, than before he suffered the reaction to the medication. I agreed to allow the dialysis, yet I feared if Keith didn't fully mentally recover, he would look at me and hate me. I couldn't bare the thought, but I wanted my son alive and well. Therefore, I had to give him the opportunity to beat this thing once again.

As it was the dialysis treatment pulled Keith through the ammonia poisoning induced coma, but the damage was done. Keith would never be mentally or physically the Keith we all knew and loved prior to receiving the Depakote. That, combined with the evidence that the demyelination seemed to be out of control as it went deeper into the brain made it all seem so hopeless. Test results would later confirm the demyelination was massive involving the left frontal, parietal and occipital lobe, the corpus callosum, and extending down to the midbrain, pons, medulla and spinal cord. I struggled with what I had previously given permission for everytime I looked at my son who vacillated in and out of reality. One moment he was coherent and the next he was hallucinating, seeing monsters, thinking he was the second coming or thinking others and myself were the devil. The family struggled with the decision to honor Keith's Advanced Directives and to allow him to go to heaven to be healed. Making the decision and having to live with it were very upsetting. Yet, I felt down deep in my heart, I knew what Keith wanted us to do. The thank you note sent to me freed our family of any mental suffering just as we had freed Keith from his physical and mental sufferings.

If you wish to honor Keith's memory I encourage you to make the same promises I did:

1. Do not let life's negative experiences make you bitter. Elton Trueblood wrote, "Life need not be easy to be joyful. Joy is not the absence of trouble but the presence of Christ."

2. Find some happiness in each day, because all those individual days will make up your life. Dr. Burkhardt, from the University of Illinois, wrote us of all the facets of Keith's personality what touched him the most was his "open, cheerful, and grateful approach to life's opportunities" because he went on to write "his attitude was contagious." To be around Keith was to experience happiness, a happiness he found in everyday living.

3. Keep your faith through all of life's trials. Without knowing all the answers for your questions trust in the wisdom and goodness of God.

4. Instead of writing a book consider writing out your Power of Attorney For Health Care to help your loved ones honor your wishes for end-of-life care. Remember, these are hard decisions, and your family will appreciate your advanced directives.

> We did it Keith, by the grace of God,
> and with the help of lots of people we
> made it through the year of the zebra,
> and we wrote the book! It is finished.

Love Always,
Mom